Copyright © 2024 by Helen Morrison

TABLE OF CONTENTS

1   INTRODCTION

Hyperthyroidism occurs when you have an overactive thyroid gland. In other words, it happens when the thyroid gland produces too much thyroid hormone. This speeds up metabolism and can affect many organs.

Common hyperthyroidism symptoms may include anxiety, nervousness, fatigue, weight loss, hand tremors, and an irregular heartbeat.

A variety of factors and conditions can cause hyperthyroidism. Prompt diagnosis and treatment can help prevent serious lifelong complications.

This book provides a detailed look at hyperthyroidism, including its symptoms, how doctors diagnose causes of hyperthyroidism, and some treatment options for hyperthyroidism.

Hyperthyroidism is also known as an overactive thyroid. The thyroid gland is located in the front of the neck. It produces thyroid hormone, which is a hormone necessary for typical metabolism.

In hyperthyroidism, the thyroid produces too much thyroid hormone. This leads to an overactive metabolism. Common hyperthyroidism symptoms include anxiety, nervousness, weight loss, and high blood pressure.

Hyperthyroidism can result from various factors, including inflammation of or a growth on the thyroid gland. Graves' disease, which is an autoimmune condition, is the most common cause of hyperthyroidism. Other causes include thyroid nodules, iodine exposure, and high levels of thyroid-stimulating hormone (TSH) from the pituitary gland.

Prompt diagnosis and treatment can lead to a good outlook. In some cases, it may also lead to curing the condition. With regular medical care and compliance with their treatment plan, many people with the condition live active, regular lives.

In some cases, however, hyperthyroidism can lead to serious, potentially life threatening symptoms and complications. These include heart arrhythmias and heart failure. Seek immediate medical care (call 911) for serious symptoms, such as chest pain, heart palpitations, or shortness of breath.

There are primary and secondary types of hyperthyroidism, which differ due to what's causing the excess production of thyroid hormone.

Primary Hyperthyroidism

In primary hyperthyroidism, a problem with the thyroid gland itself results in the overproduction of thyroid hormones.

Laboratory tests will show too much triiodothyronine (T3) and thyroxine (T4) two of the main hormones that your thyroid produces. Causes of primary hyperthyroidism include:

- Graves' Disease
- Toxic multinodular goiter

- Toxic adenoma

- Thyroid inflammation (thyroiditis)

Secondary Hyperthyroidism

In secondary hyperthyroidism, the thyroid gland itself is normal, but something is causing it to make too much thyroid hormone. This is usually due to an excess of thyroid hormone secretion from the brain. However, in some cases, cancers elsewhere in the body can produce hormones that look similar to thyroid hormone, causing an excess of T3 and T4. Secondary hyperthyroidism can occur as a result of:

- Pituitary adenoma (brain tumor)

- Choriocarcinoma (tumor in the uterus)

- Ovarian cancer

- Testicular cancer

2.2 What are the Symptoms of Hyperthyroidism?

Hyperthyroidism symptoms are the result of an overactive metabolism.

Common symptoms include:

- anxiety, nervousness, and irritability
- diarrhea
- difficulty sleeping
- extremely smooth skin
- changes in the nails
- eye symptoms (thyroid eye disease), such as bulging eyes, eye puffiness, light sensitivity, and an intense stare
- swelling of the thyroid gland in the front of the neck (a goiter)

- increased appetite but unexpected weight loss
- increased sensitivity to heat
- muscle weakness and fatigue
- shaky hands or tremors
- sweating

2.3 WHAT CAUSES HYPERTHYROIDISM?

Hyperthyroidism occurs when the thyroid gland is overactive and produces too much thyroid hormone. A variety of conditions can stimulate the thyroid gland to make too much thyroid hormone.

Some causes of hyperthyroidism include:

- Autoimmune thyroid disease: This is also known as Graves' disease, and it occurs when the immune system makes a typical autoantibodies that attach to thyroid gland cells and stimulate them to secrete excess thyroid hormone. This is the most common cause of hyperthyroidism.

- Excess levels of TSH: This occurs when the pituitary gland produces too much TSH.

- Iodine exposure: The thyroid uses iodine to produce thyroid hormone. Consuming too much iodine can cause hyperthyroidism.

- Overactive thyroid nodule: This noncancerous cyst grows on the thyroid gland and produces additional thyroid hormone. This more commonly affects older adults.

- Thyroiditis: This refers to inflammation of the thyroid gland due to a viral infection. It may also develop after giving birth (postpartum thyroiditis).

- High dosages of thyroid hormone medications: If you are taking thyroid hormone medications for hypothyroidism, you should have your thyroid hormone levels checked at least once per year to determine if the dosage needs adjusting. Some medications can interact with thyroid hormone medications, so it is important to check with your doctor about all medications and supplements you take.

2.4 HYPERTHYROIDISM VS. HYPOTHYROIDISM

The thyroid gland can become overactive or underactive. An underactive thyroid makes less thyroid hormone than the body requires. This is called hypothyroidism.

Like hyperthyroidism, the most common cause of hypothyroidism is an autoimmune condition. However, with autoimmune hypothyroidism (Hashimoto's thyroiditis), the body makes antibodies that attack the thyroid gland. This causes inflammation that disrupts the ability of the thyroid gland to make hormones.

Subclinical vs. overt hyperthyroidism

Subclinical hyperthyroidism means that you have low or undetectable TSH with normal free thyroxine (T3) and total or free triiodothyronine (T4) levels.

Overt hyperthyroidism is defined by low or undetectable TSH with high free T3 or high free T4 levels.

2.4.1 What are the risk factors for hyperthyroidism?

Females are more likely than males to develop hyperthyroidism. However, several other factors increase the risk of developing the condition. Not all people who are at risk of hyperthyroidism will develop it.

Risk factors include:

- being assigned female at birth
- being 40 years or younger or 60 years or older
- having certain common viral infections
- receiving particular drug treatments, such as certain cancer and AIDS therapies
- having a family history of thyroid disease, including Graves' disease
- having a history of autoimmune conditions

- having iodine exposure, including from foods containing iodine and some heart medications

- having a recent pregnancy

- taking too high a dosage of thyroid replacement hormone

- sustaining trauma or an injury to the thyroid

- having other health conditions, including:

- diabetes

- pernicious anemia (from a vitamin B12 deficiency)

- adrenal insufficiency (reduced production of certain hormones)

2.5   HOW DO YOU PREVENT HYPERTHYROIDISM?

In general, it is not possible to prevent hyperthyroidism. Most of the risk factors and causes are not avoidable.

If you take thyroid replacement hormone for an underactive thyroid, regular monitoring will help keep your levels in the appropriate range.

If you have risk factors for hyperthyroidism, talk with your doctor about how to recognize early symptoms.

2.6 HOW DO DOCTORS DIAGNOSE HYPERTHYROIDISM?

To diagnose hyperthyroidism, your doctor will take a medical history, perform an exam, and order thyroid tests.

During the exam, your doctor will feel the thyroid gland in your neck. They may also test your reflexes, check your pulse, and examine your eyes and skin. You may also need to extend your arms and hands so that your doctor can see if your hands are steady.

Tests to diagnose thyroid disease, including hyperthyroidism, include:

- Blood tests: These tests measure the amount of TSH, T4, T3, and thyroid antibodies.
- Thyroid scan: This imaging exam uses a radioactive injection to check how much iodine your thyroid absorbs. This highlights nonfunctioning areas of the thyroid gland. This is also known as a radioiodine uptake test.
- Thyroid ultrasound: This imaging exam looks for thyroid nodules without using radiation.

Your doctor may also ask you several questions about your symptoms, medical history, and any medications you take. These questions may include:

- What symptoms are you experiencing?

- When did your symptoms begin?

- Are your symptoms constant, or do they come and go?

- What, if anything, seems to make your symptoms better or worse?

- Do you have a family history of thyroid disease?

- What other medical conditions do you have?

- What medications do you take?

- Have you recently been pregnant or given birth?

- How do you treat hyperthyroidism?

Prompt diagnosis and treatment of an overactive thyroid can return thyroid hormone to appropriate levels. Treating hyperthyroidism is important to relieve symptoms and prevent health problems.

Doctors recommend treatments depending on how severe your symptoms are and what is causing your hyperthyroidism.

Hyperthyroidism treatment includes:

- Beta-blockers: These drugs can minimize some of the symptoms, such as a rapid heart rate and anxiety.

- Antithyroid or hyperthyroidism medication: This type of therapy decreases the overproduction of thyroid hormone. In some cases, antithyroid medications may even cure hyperthyroidism.

- Thyroid surgery: This procedure removes part or most of the overactive thyroid gland. If a surgeon removes part of the thyroid, thyroid hormone levels may return to normal, curing the condition. If they remove the entire thyroid, it results in an underactive thyroid, and you will need lifelong thyroid hormone replacement.

- Radioactive iodine: Swallowing radioactive iodine can reduce overactivity and overproduction of thyroid hormone. This treatment can also result in underactive thyroid and the need for lifelong thyroid hormone replacement. It may also lead to normalized thyroid hormone levels.

- Hypothyroidism medication adjustments: This involves testing levels of thyroid hormone in the blood and lowering the dosage of thyroid hormone medications used to treat hypothyroidism.

2.7   HOW DOES HYPERTHYROIDISM AFFECT QUALITY OF LIFE?

The thyroid gland influences just about every bodily function. When there is a problem with this gland, your whole body can feel the effects. You may experience reductions in physical, mental, and emotional well-being.

All of this can contribute to decreases in quality of life (QoL). Eye symptoms, fatigue, depression, and anxiety can all contribute to decreased QoL in hyperthyroidism.

Researchers have studied the effect that treatments have on improving QoL for people with Graves' hypothyroidism. They compared people who received radioiodine therapy with those who underwent surgery (thyroidectomy) and took antithyroid drugs.

Around 6–10 years later, people with Graves' hypothyroidism had lower QoL regardless of treatment compared with people in general. People who received radioiodine treatment reported worse thyroid-related QoL than people who underwent surgery and took antithyroid drugs.

If you are considering treatment options, talk with your doctor about QoL issues. Be sure to ask about the latest research in this area and what you can expect with treatment.

2.8 WHAT ARE THE POTENTIAL COMPLICATIONS OF HYPERTHYROIDISM?

Complications of untreated hyperthyroidism can be serious. Some can even be life threatening. You can help reduce the risk of serious complications by following your treatment plan.

Complications of untreated hyperthyroidism include:

- angina, heart failure, or hypertension
- anxiety and depression
- eye and vision problems (thyroid eye disease), such as bulging eyes, puffy eyes, chronic eye irritation, and vision changes
- hair loss

- an irregular heartbeat, including cardiac arrhythmias, heart palpitations, and a rapid heart rate

- osteoporosis and muscle weakness

- thyrotoxic crisis, which is an acute severe worsening of symptoms that can be life threatening

- unintended weight loss

3 DOES HYPERTHYROIDISM CAUSE WEIGHT GAIN?

Hyperthyroidism occurs when your thyroid makes too much thyroid hormone. Typically, hyperthyroidism causes weight loss, but in some cases, it can cause weight gain.

Your thyroid is a butterfly-shaped gland in your neck. Thyroid hormone affects how your body uses energy, also known as metabolism. Causes of hyperthyroidism include Graves' disease, thyroid inflammation, or an overactive thyroid nodule.

Read on to learn how hyperthyroidism may cause weight gain. This book also discusses when to see a doctor, how to address weight gain from hyperthyroidism, and answers some frequently asked questions.

3.1 HOW DOES HYPERTHYROIDISM AFFECT YOUR WEIGHT?

The hormones your thyroid gland secretes play a significant role in weight management, and specifically, how your body uses energy. A change in your thyroid hormone level alters your resting metabolic rate (RMR), which is how many calories your body uses when resting.

Hyperthyroidism is more common in people who were assigned female at birth and those over 60 years of age. About 1 in 100 people in the United States over the age of 12 have hyperthyroidism.

When you have more thyroid hormone, as in hyperthyroidism, your RMR increases and causes your body to burn more calories.

In contrast, when you have less thyroid hormone, as in hypothyroidism, your RMR decreases, and your body does not burn as many calories.

3.2   How can hyperthyroidism cause weight gain?

While most people lose weight when they have hyperthyroidism, according to a 2019 study, about 10% can gain weight. This may be due to eating more because of a larger appetite, hyperthyroidism treatments, and thyroid inflammation.

Increased appetite

If you have hyperthyroidism, you may feel more hungry because of your increased RMR. Some people with hyperthyroidism start eating more food to fulfill their hunger, leading to weight gain.

To help you feel more satiated, consider foods that provide nutrients and vitamins. The Centers for Disease Control and Prevention (CDC) recommends focusing on lean proteins and a variety of fruits and vegetables. It also recommends avoiding or limiting processed foods and baked goods containing white flour and sugar.

Hyperthyroidism treatment

Treating your hyperthyroidism depends on the underlying cause. The goal is to bring your thyroid hormone back to a normal level. Your doctor may prescribe antithyroid medications, radioiodine, or suggest you have all or part of your thyroid removed.

When you bring your thyroid hormone back to normal, you may experience some weight gain due to your RMR slowing down. You may need to make lifestyle changes such as physically moving more and eating fewer calories to maintain a moderate weight.

Thyroiditis

Thyroiditis is when your immune system attacks your thyroid gland and causes inflammation. One of the most common causes of thyroiditis is Hashimoto's disease, an autoimmune condition. Some people with Graves' disease also have antibodies for Hashimoto's disease.

When Hashimoto's disease attacks the thyroid gland, it can damage it and cause hypothyroidism. If this occurs, you have less circulating thyroid hormone and a decreased RMR. These conditions may cause weight gain.

Other symptoms of Hashimoto's disease include:

- enlarged thyroid gland
- feeling cold
- constipation
- fatigue
- heavy menstrual cycles
- Talk with your doctor if you experience weight gain along with these other symptoms. Your doctor may suggest making changes to your treatment plan.

When should you see a doctor for weight gain with hyperthyroidism?

Most of the time, a little weight gain with hyperthyroidism is not a concern, especially if you are beginning treatment.

You may have been in a hyperthyroid state for some time and lost weight due to excessive thyroid hormone. Now that your hormones are leveling out, you may notice some weight gain.

However, if you notice you are consistently increasing in weight and are experiencing symptoms of Hashimoto's disease, you may want to consider speaking with your doctor.

Your doctor can check your thyroid hormone levels and other complications. When your doctor discovers the cause of the weight gain, they can alter your treatment plan accordingly.

How can you address weight gain from hyperthyroidism?

The first step to safely addressing your weight gain from hyperthyroidism is understanding that your previous weight loss was temporary due to an overactive thyroid. Treatment to stabilize your hormone levels may cause weight gain, which is to be expected.

You may need to rethink your eating habits. Work with your doctor or a certified nutritionist on eating habits that are sustainable for you. They can help you understand how many calories you need daily and which foods to focus on. They can also give guidelines on which foods to limit or avoid.

Having your doctor check your thyroid hormones regularly is a good idea. At the beginning of treatment, it is possible to overtreat hormone imbalance.. At the beginning of treatment, it is possible to overtreat hormone imbalance. This can cause hypothyroid or underactive thyroid conditions. Checking your levels frequently can help your doctor adjust treatment as needed.

4 HYPERTHYROIDISM DIET: FOODS TO EAT, LIMIT, AND AVOID

Low-iodine foods such as fruits, vegetables, and unsalted nuts may be beneficial if you have hyperthyroidism. Foods to avoid or limit include dairy, eggs, and pasta.

Hyperthyroidism is a condition in which there's too much thyroid hormone in your body. Graves' disease, an autoimmune condition, can cause hyperthyroidism. Common symptoms include weight loss, fast heartbeat, and trouble sleeping.

There is a lack of extensive human studies on a specific diet for hyperthyroidism. Most recommendations for foods to include, limit, or avoid are based on animal studies or single-case reports. While specific diets are not generally part of clinical treatment for hyperthyroidism, some people may find it helps manage their symptoms.

The word "diet" can have many meanings. This article uses the term "diet" to refer to an eating lifestyle rather than a temporary change in how you eat.

How does diet affect hyperthyroidism?

Though no dietary cure for hyperthyroidism exists, some foods may enhance symptoms while others ease them.

Iodine is a nutrient your thyroid uses to make more thyroid hormones. Hyperthyroidism means the thyroid is producing too much thyroid hormone. In this case, limiting or avoiding foods that contain high levels of iodine may be a good idea.

Foods that can be beneficial if you have hyperthyroidism include cruciferous vegetables, like broccoli and cabbage, and foods with soy or specific vitamins. These help inhibit thyroid hormone production.

4.1 WHAT FOODS SHOULD YOU EAT WITH HYPERTHYROIDISM?

Several foods may help ease and manage symptoms of hyperthyroidism.

Low-iodine foods

Iodine is a natural element that some foods have. Foods high in iodine may worsen symptoms, so limiting or avoiding them is a good idea. Talk with a healthcare professional about how much iodine you should limit.

Foods that are low in iodine include:

- spices and herbs
- non-iodized salt
- vegetable oils
- egg whites
- fresh or frozen fruits and vegetables
- sweeteners such as maple syrup, honey, and sugar
- unsalted nuts and nut butter
- jams or jellies
- moderate portions of beef, poultry, and lamb
- lemonade

Cruciferous vegetables

According to experts, cruciferous vegetables contain compounds that may decrease the production of thyroid hormones.

Cruciferous vegetables include:

- broccoli and cauliflower
- brussels sprouts
- cabbage
- arugula
- bok choy
- kale
- watercress
- turnip
- radish
- rutabaga

Foods containing selenium

Selenium is a micronutrient that may help improve thyroid health.

Selenium is found in:

- brazil nuts

- shellfish

- fortified cereals

- whole wheat bread

- beans and lentils

- Beef and poultry are good sources of selenium but contain iodine. Consider smaller portions of these items if you have hyperthyroidism.

Foods containing iron

Iron deficiency anemia often accompanies hyperthyroidism. Many people with hyperthyroidism require supplementation with iron.

Foods high in iron include:

- raisins

- fortified cereals

- spinach

- Poultry, oysters, and fish contain iron. However, they can also contain iodine. Be sure to follow a healthcare professional's recommendations on how much iodine is safe to eat daily.

Foods containing calcium and vitamin D

Thyroid hormones are essential for bone health. People with hyperthyroidism frequently experience decreased bone density, which leads to osteoporosis. Foods that are rich in calcium to consider adding to your meals are:

- milk
- cheese
- yogurt
- calcium-fortified orange juice
- broccoli

- kale
- bok choy

Vitamin D deficiency is also common among people with hyperthyroidism. You can get vitamin D through safe sun exposure to your skin. However, you may also need supplementation to increase your levels.

Because foods are not a great source of vitamin D, talk with a healthcare professional about which vitamin D supplement they recommend. Some foods are fortified with vitamin D, however.

Those foods include:

- fortified milk
- fortified cereals
- fortified yogurts

4.2 WHAT FOODS SHOULD YOU AVOID WITH HYPERTHYROIDISM?

If you have hyperthyroidism, avoid or limit the following foods.

Iodine-rich foods

The mineral iodine helps increase how much hormone your thyroid produces. Iodine-rich foods include:

- seaweed or kelp
- cod fish
- bread enriched with iodine
- oysters
- dairy products
- iodized salt
- pasta

- eggs

- shrimp

- tuna

Soy

Soy contains compounds that may interfere with thyroid function and cause your thyroid to grow. Limiting or avoiding foods high in soy is a good idea if you have hyperthyroidism.

These foods include:

- edamame

- meat alternatives

- soy milk

- soy nuts

- soy sauce

- tofu

- soybeans

Gluten

People with hyperthyroidism caused by Graves' disease are at higher risk of celiac disease. Celiac disease is an autoimmune condition that causes inflammation of the intestines. Gluten is a protein found in wheat that people with celiac disease cannot digest.

If you have hyperthyroidism and experience gastrointestinal discomfort, you may want to talk with a healthcare professional about limiting or avoiding foods with gluten. These include:

- pasta
- baked goods
- cereal

- crackers

- soups that contain pasta or flour

- beer

- gravy

Caffeine

Caffeine intake could worsen several symptoms of hyperthyroidism, such as insomnia, fast heartbeat, and hand tremors.

Foods and beverages high in caffeine include:

- coffee

- black tea

- dark chocolate

- regular soda

- energy drinks

5   HYPERTHYROIDISM DIET RECIPES

5.1   BREAKFAST

5.2   BREAKFAST SMOOTHIE

Ingredients

4 ounces pure pomegranate juice, no sugar added

1 cup mixed berries

1 small banana

½ cup apple juice, no sugar added

1 tablespoon flaxseeds

Ice cubes

Cooking Instructions

Place all the ingredients in a blender and fill with ice. Puree on high speed until smooth. Divide between two tall glasses and serve immediately with a straw.

Ingredients

For the crêpes:

1 cup sifted flour

2 extra-large eggs, beaten

1 tablespoon honey, warmed in the microwave

2 tablespoons unsalted butter, melted

Pinch salt

1 cup low-fat milk

2 cups fresh raspberries

For the filling:

1½ cups low-fat cottage cheese

¼ cup low-fat sour cream

1 tablespoon honey, warmed in the microwave

Pinch salt

Cooking Instructions

For the filling: Mix in a bowl the cottage cheese, sour cream, honey, and salt. Refrigerate until use.

Place 1 cup of the raspberries in a blender and reduce to a sauce. Pass through a sieve to remove seeds and refrigerate until use.

For the crêpes: Place the flour in a bowl. Blend in the eggs, honey, salt, and melted butter. Slowly whisk in the milk. Let the batter rest for 30 minutes. Before use, add a little water to thin out the batter. Heat a nonstick pan or crêpe pan over medium heat. Soak a small piece of paper towel in vegetable oil and swirl quickly over the pan. Add enough batter and swirl to cover the entire bottom. Cook until golden brown and remove from heat. Do not cook the other side. Repeat until all the batter has been used.

Place the golden brown side of the crêpes side up. Divide the filling among the center length of the crêpes. Roll a bit, tuck both edges, and finish rolling to retain all the filling inside the crêpes. Cook the crêpes over medium heat in a greased skillet until golden brown on all sides. Serve immediately with the raspberry coulis and the remaining raspberries.

5.4   FRENCH TOAST WITH ORANGE SLICES

Ingredients

3 eggs

2/3 cup low-fat milk

1½ teaspoons orange extract

Pinch salt

8 slices whole wheat bread

Vegetable oil

4 tablespoons maple syrup

2 oranges, peeled and sliced

Cooking Instructions

Beat together the eggs, milk, orange extract, and salt. Dip the bread slices in the mixture. Soak them well.

Preheat two large skillets or a griddle with a little vegetable oil. Add the bread slices and brown on both sides. Serve immediately with maple syrup and orange slices.

5.5 GRANOLA WITH BANANA, APPLE, AND WALNUT

Ingredients

½ cup granola

½ cup low-fat milk

¼ small banana, peeled and sliced

¼ medium apple, peeled, cored, and diced

1 teaspoon chopped walnuts

Cooking Instructions

Mix the granola with the milk. Add the banana, apples, and walnuts, and serve immediately.

5.6 ORANGE WHEAT MUFFINS WITH CREAM CHEESE

Ingredients

1 cup unbleached all-purpose flour

½ cup whole wheat flour

½ cup flaxseed meal

⅓ cup honey

1 teaspoon baking soda

1 tablespoon baking powder

¼ teaspoon salt

1 teaspoon orange extract

1 teaspoon orange zest

2 large eggs

2 tablespoons canola oil

½ cup pumpkin puree (organic can)

1 cup plain low-fat yogurt

12 tablespoons low-fat cream cheese

12 teaspoons pumpkin seeds

Pumpkin pie spices or cinnamon to taste (optional)

Cooking Instructions

Preheat the oven to 375°F.

Blend the flours, flaxseed meal, honey, baking soda, baking powder, and salt in a mixing bowl. Blend in the orange extract, orange zest, canola oil, eggs, pumpkin puree, yogurt, and mix well. Fill muffin pan and bake for 25 minutes or until cooked through and golden brown.

Top each muffin with 1 tablespoon of low-fat cream cheese. Sprinkle spices or cinnamon, pumpkin seeds, and serve immediately.

5.7   RYE BREAD WITH CREAM CHEESE AND SALMON

Ingredients

1½ tablespoons low-fat cream cheese

1 slice rye bread

1 slice smoked salmon (about ¾ ounces)

Lemon juice

Cooking Instructions

Spread the cream cheese over the bread. Add the smoked salmon, sprinkle a little lemon juice, and serve immediately.

5.8   SCRAMBLED EGGS WITH MUSHROOMS AND ONIONS

Ingredients

1 teaspoon olive oil

½ small yellow onion, chopped (about 2 ounces)

4 white mushrooms, sliced (about 4 ounces)

1 garlic clove, minced (optional)

1 tablespoon freshly minced basil

4 eggs

1 tablespoon low-fat milk

Salt and pepper to taste

Cooking Instructions

Heat the oil in a nonstick pan over medium heat. Add the onion and sauté until translucent. Add the garlic, mushrooms, and sauté until mushrooms are cooked through. Beat the eggs with the milk in a bowl. Add the basil and season to taste. Pour the mixture over the vegetables. Cook over medium heat, stirring and scraping the bottom and sides of the pan constantly with a wooden spoon. As soon as the eggs begin to set, remove from heat, continue to stir for a few seconds, and serve immediately.

5.9 Strawberry, Pomegranate, and Spinach Smoothie

Ingredients

2 cups strawberries (about 10 ounces)

1 bunch fresh spinach (at least 2 cups)

1 small banana

1 pomegranate

1 tablespoon flaxseeds

Ice cubes

Cooking Instructions

De-seed the pomegranate. Place the seeds in a blender and add the remaining ingredients. Fill with ice and puree on high speed until smooth. Divide between two tall glasses and serve immediately with a straw.

5.10 Cream of Millet

Ingredients

1 cup low-fat rice or almond milk

Small pinch salt

1 teaspoon pumpkin pie spices (optional)

¼ cup pearl millet

2 teaspoons slivered almonds

2 teaspoons maple syrup

½ peach, peeled, seeded, and diced

1 teaspoon flaxseed oil

Cooking Instructions

Warm the milk, salt, and pumpkin pie spices over medium heat in a small saucepan. Wash the millet a couple of times and drain well. Place the millet in another pan over medium heat. Add the almonds and the warm flavored milk. Reduce heat and simmer for 20 minutes or until all the liquid is absorbed.

Transfer to a serving bowl and mix in the maple syrup. Top with the fruits, drizzle flaxseed oil, and serve immediately.

5.11 HOMEMADE GRANOLA

Ingredients

¼ cup honey

¼ cup grapeseed oil

2 teaspoons cinnamon

1 teaspoon almond extract

1 teaspoon orange extract

3½ cups rolled oats

¼ cup slivered almonds

¼ cup chopped walnuts

Cooking Instructions

Preheat the oven to 350°F. In a bowl, mix the honey, spices, oil, and extracts. Stir in the oats and nuts. Mix well and spread over a greased cookie sheet. Bake for 10 minutes. Stir and continue to bake for another 10 minutes, or until golden brown. Cool completely and break apart. Store in an airtight container away from heat.

You may substitute the honey with agave nectar. Enjoy with low-fat soy milk, low-fat rice milk, low-fat almond milk, low-fat milk, low-fat plain yogurt, or a mix of low-fat milk and low-fat plain yogurt. Top with your favorite fruits for added nutritional values.

Add 1 teaspoon freshly ground flaxseeds per serving before serving.

5.12   MUESLI WITH DRIED FRUIT AND NUTS

Ingredients

½ cup muesli cereal

½ cup low-fat rice or almond milk

1 tablespoon mixed dried berries

1 tablespoon raisins

1 teaspoon slivered or sliced almonds

1 teaspoon chopped walnuts

Cooking Instructions

In a bowl, mix the cereal with the milk. If too thick, add a little more milk to thin out. Top with the mixed dried berries, raisins, almonds, and walnuts, and serve immediately.

5.13 Oat Bran–Flax Muffin

Ingredients

1 cup unbleached all-purpose flour

½ cup oat bran flour

½ cup flaxseed meal

½ cup brown sugar

1½ teaspoons baking soda

1 teaspoon baking powder

¼ teaspoon salt

1½ tablespoons ground cinnamon

1 teaspoon ground ginger

1¼ cups shredded peeled carrots

2 medium apples, peeled, cored, and finely diced

¾ cup walnuts, chopped

¾ cup dried berries and raisins blend (about equal amount of each)

¼ cup canola oil

1 teaspoon vanilla extract

2 eggs, mixed

½ cup rice or almond milk

Cooking Instructions

Preheat the oven to 350°F.

In a bowl, blend the flours, flaxseed meal, brown sugar, baking soda, baking powder, salt, cinnamon, and ginger. Mix in the carrots, apples, walnuts, and berry-raisin blend. Add the oil, vanilla, eggs (or banana and apple sauce mixture), and milk, and mix until incorporated. Grease the muffin tin with canola oil. Divide mix among the 12 cups of a muffin tin and bake between 20 to 25 minutes.

You can substitute the eggs with equal parts mashed banana and apple sauce, equaling the same net weight as the eggs.

5.14 Whole Grain Bread with Almond Butter, Pears, and Walnuts

Ingredients

1 tablespoon almond butter

1 slice whole grain bread

½ medium pear, peeled, cored, and sliced

½ teaspoon chopped walnuts

Cooking Instructions

Spread the almond butter over the bread. Layer the pear slices on top, sprinkle with walnuts, and serve immediately.

5.15 Grapefruit and Crabmeat Salad

Ingredients

1 large pink grapefruit (about 16 ounces grapefruit)

8 ounces crabmeat portions, excess water removed

2 tablespoons low-fat canola mayonnaise

1 cup lettuce, shredded

1 tablespoon freshly minced cilantro

Chili powder to taste

Salt and pepper to taste

Cooking Instructions

Place the crabmeat in a bowl.

Cut the grapefruit in half. Insert a thin knife all around the skin to loosen up the flesh. Separate the flesh from the skin and place it on a cutting board. Dice the flesh small and transfer to the crabmeat bowl. Add mayonnaise, chili powder, cilantro, and season to taste. Cover with plastic wrap and refrigerate for half an hour.

Equally divide the lettuce in two plates and top with the prepared grapefruit crabmeat salad.

5.16 Greek Salad with Cod

Ingredients

4 tablespoons vinaigrette

1 teaspoon freshly minced oregano

4 cups mixed greens

1 large cucumber, peeled, seeded, and sliced (about 12 ounces)

2 large tomatoes, sliced (about 12 ounces)

½ small red onion, sliced (about 2 ounces)

1 medium red bell pepper, seeded, ribs removed, and sliced (about 6 ounces)

¼ cup black olives

4 tablespoons feta cheese

Four 4-ounce cooked cod fillets

Salt and pepper to taste

Cooking instructions

Mix the vinaigrette with the oregano and set aside.

Divide the mixed greens, cucumber, tomatoes, red onion, bell pepper, black olives, and feta cheese among 4 plates. Top with the fish fillet and season with salt and pepper. Drizzle with the vinaigrette and serve immediately.

5.17 Smoked Salmon, Potato, and Watercress Salad

Ingredients

12 ounces smoked salmon, diced

3 cooked potatoes, sliced (about 1 pound)

1 bunch watercress

1 cup cooked green beans

1 hardboiled egg, chopped (or 2 egg whites for less cholesterol)

2 tablespoons white wine vinegar

4 tablespoons olive oil

1 teaspoon Dijon mustard

1 tablespoon minced shallots

2 tablespoons minced salad herbs

Salt and pepper to taste

Cooking Instructions

Mix the vinegar, mustard, and shallots in a bowl. Whisk in the olive oil, 1 tablespoon of minced herbs, and season to taste.

Mix half of the dressing with the potatoes. Mix the remaining dressing with the watercress. Divide the watercress among four plates. Top with the potatoes, broccoli, and salmon. Sprinkle with the chopped egg, remaining minced herbs, and serve immediately.

5.18 Sugar Snap Peas and Tuna Salad

Ingredients

For the salad:

4 ounces Boston lettuce

1½ cans tuna in water, strained (9 ounces)

1 large carrot, thinly sliced (about 4 ounces)

2 large tomatoes, seeded and diced

1 cup fresh sugar snap peas (about 4 ounces)

Salt and pepper to taste

For the dressing:

1 shallot, minced

1 garlic clove, minced (optional)

3 tablespoons lemon juice

3 tablespoons olive oil

2 tablespoons salad herbs

Salt and pepper to taste

Cooking Instructions

Heat a steamer and add the sugar snap peas. Cook for 2 minutes. Add the carrots and continue to steam for 2 minutes or until desired doneness. In a bowl, mix the shallot, garlic, lemon juice, oil, 1 tablespoon of herbs, and season to taste. In a large bowl mix the lettuce with half of the dressing. Add the tuna, tomatoes, carrot slices, and sugar snap peas. Sprinkle with the remaining herbs and dressing before serving.

5.19 TOMATO, MOZZARELLA, AND BASIL SALAD

Ingredients

6 large tomatoes, sliced (about 2¼ pounds)

1 shallot, minced

1 garlic clove, minced (optional)

4 tablespoons olive oil

2 tablespoons white wine or apple cider vinegar

8 fresh basil leaves

8 ounces fresh mozzarella cheese, sliced

Cooking Instructions

Spread the tomatoes over a large platter. Sprinkle with salt and set aside for 20 minutes. Mince half the basil leaves and set aside. Shred the remaining leaves and set aside.

Mix the shallot, garlic, and vinegar in a bowl. Whisk in the oil, the minced basil, and season to taste.

Transfer the tomatoes to another serving platter. Alternate a tomato slice and mozzarella slice. Spread the shredded basil, pour the dressing over, and serve immediately.

5.20 CARROT AND APPLE SOUP

Ingredients

5 large carrots, peeled and sliced (about 20 ounces)

1 large Golden Delicious apple, peeled and quartered (about 6 ounces)

1 medium onion, peeled and quartered (about 6 ounces)

4 cups gluten-free chicken stock (low-fat and low-sodium)

1 bouquet garni

¼ teaspoon ground ginger

Salt and pepper to taste

Cooking Instructions

Place the carrots, apple, onion, stock, bouquet garni, and ginger in a large pan. Bring to boil over medium heat. Reduce heat, cover, and simmer until the vegetables are cooked through, 10 to 15 minutes. Transfer to a blender and puree with enough of the liquid to obtain a soup consistency. Season with salt and pepper and serve immediately.

5.21 Cod and Corn Chowder

Ingredients

2 teaspoons grapeseed oil

1 medium onion, diced (about 6 ounces)

1 medium carrot, diced (about 3 ounces)

1 large celery stalk, diced (about 2 ounces)

2 medium potatoes, peeled and diced (about 12 ounces)

Corn kernels from 2 corn ears

2 cups vegetable stock (low-fat and low-sodium)

1 cup low-fat milk

1 pound cod fish fillets, diced

2 tablespoons freshly minced parsley

Salt and pepper to taste

Cooking Instructions

Heat the oil in a saucepan over high heat. Add the onion and sauté until translucent. Add the carrot, celery, potatoes, stock, and bring to a boil. Reduce heat and simmer for 15 minutes. Mash the potato with a fork and continue to reduce until you obtain a creamy texture. Add the corn, milk, fish, parsley, and bring to a boil. Continue to simmer for another 5 minutes. Adjust seasoning and serve immediately.

French Onion Soup

Ingredients

2 tablespoons grapeseed oil

3 large onions, thinly sliced (about 1½ pounds)

2 tablespoons Cognac (optional)

2 tablespoons flour

6 to 7 cups beef stock (low-fat and low-sodium)

¾ cup Swiss cheese or Gruyère, shredded (about 6 ounces)

Salt and pepper to taste

Cooking Instructions

Heat the oil in a large pan over medium heat. Add the onions and cook until golden brown. Stir occasionally to avoid burning. This will take up to 20 minutes. Carefully add the cognac and flambé (optional). Sprinkle with the flour and mix well. Add the beef stock and bring to a boil over high heat. Reduce heat and simmer for 20 to 25 minutes. Skim any foam or fat that may rise to the surface. Adjust seasonings and serve immediately with the cheese.

5.22 OYSTER STEW

Ingredients

2 cups low-fat milk

½ tablespoon olive oil

½ quart oysters

1 tablespoon parsley

Salt and pepper to taste

Cornstarch mixed with a little water

Cooking Instructions

Scald the milk in a saucepan over medium heat. Thicken with a little cornstarch to obtain a sauce consistency. Carefully open the oysters and transfer their liquid to a bowl. Remove flesh and add to a pan. Add the olive oil and quickly sauté under medium heat. Add the liquid and simmer (do not boil) until the edges begin to curl. Add the hot milk, parsley, and season to taste. Bring to a simmer (do not boil) and serve immediately.

5.23 PUMPKIN SOUP

Ingredients

1 (3 pound) pumpkin

1 teaspoon olive oil

2 large onions, sliced (about 1 pound)

1 garlic clove, minced (optional)

6 cups chicken stock (low-fat and low-sodium)

2 cups low-fat milk

2 fresh sage leaves

3 tablespoons low-fat Greek yogurt

2 tablespoons pumpkin seeds

Salt and pepper to taste

Cooking Instructions

Peel the pumpkin and cut the flesh into medium cubes.

Heat the oil in a large pan over high heat. Add the onions and sauté until translucent. Add the pumpkin, garlic, stock, milk, and sage, and bring to a boil. Reduce heat, cover, and simmer for 30 minutes. Transfer to a blender and puree with enough of the liquid to obtain a creamy consistency. Return to the pan, then season with salt and pepper. Before serving, add the yogurt and garnish with the pumpkin seeds.

5.24 ARTICHOKE AND FAVA BEAN SALAD

Ingredients

For the vinaigrette:

2 shallots, minced

1 large garlic clove, minced

1 teaspoon Dijon mustard

4 tablespoons balsamic vinegar

6 tablespoons olive oil

2 tablespoons flaxseed oil (or olive oil, if flaxseed oil unavailable)

3 tablespoons salad herbs

Salt and pepper to taste

For the salad:

4 ounces Boston lettuce

8 ounces cooked fava beans

1 cup cooked artichoke hearts

8 cherry tomatoes

4 ounces feta cheese, cut into 1-inch cubes

4 teaspoons slivered almonds

Cooking Instructions

For the vinaigrette: In a bowl, mix the shallots, garlic, mustard, and vinegar. Slowly whisk in the oils. Add the herbs and season with salt and pepper. For the salad: Line a serving platter with the lettuce. Spread the fava beans, artichokes hearts, and tomatoes on top of the lettuce. Drizzle with the vinaigrette. Add the feta cheese and almonds, and serve immediately.

5.25 BEETS WITH WALNUTS

Ingredients

For the salad:

2 large beets (about 20 ounces)

¼ cup walnuts, chopped

For the dressing:

1 small shallot, minced

1 large garlic clove, minced (optional)

1 teaspoon Dijon mustard

1½ tablespoons lemon juice

1 tablespoon minced fresh parsley

3 tablespoons walnut oil

Salt and pepper to taste

Cooking Instructions

For the salad: Place the beets in a large pan, cover with water, and bring to a boil over high heat. Reduce heat, cover, and simmer for 30 minutes or until cooked through. Drain and cool. Peel, slice, and place in a serving bowl.

For the dressing: In a bowl, mix the shallot, garlic, mustard, lemon juice, and parsley. Blend in the oil and season with salt and pepper.

Mix the beets with the dressing, sprinkle the walnuts over, and serve immediately.

5.26 Four Bean Salad

Ingredients

For the dressing:

1 large garlic clove, minced

2 tablespoons olive oil

4 tablespoons apple cider vinegar

2 tablespoons freshly minced salad herbs

Salt and pepper to taste

For the salad:

4 ounces dried garbanzo beans

4 ounces dried black beans

4 ounces dried red beans

4 ounces green beans

¼ small red onion, diced (about 1 ounce)

Salt

Cooking Instructions

For the dressing: In a bowl, mix the garlic, oil, vinegar, and salad herbs, and season with salt and pepper.

For the salad: Cook the garbanzo, black, and red beans separately, following package instructions. (Generally, it takes 30 to 45 minutes to cook them.) Cover the green beans with water in a pan, add a little salt, and bring to boil over high heat. Cook to desired tenderness. Drain and place immediately in ice-cold water to stop the cooking process. Drain and pat dry. In a large bowl, place all the beans and red onion, add the dressing, and adjust seasonings. Refrigerate for an hour before serving.

5.27 Leeks with Walnut Vinaigrette

Ingredients

For the salad:

8 small leeks

For the vinaigrette:

1 large garlic clove, minced

1 large shallot, minced

¼ cup walnuts, finely chopped

1 teaspoon Dijon mustard

2 tablespoons tarragon vinegar

4 tablespoons walnut oil

2 tablespoons olive oil

1 tablespoon minced fresh chives

1 tablespoon minced fresh parsley

Salt alt and pepper to taste

Cooking Instructions

For the vinaigrette: In a bowl mix the garlic, shallot, walnuts, mustard, and vinegar. Slowly whisk in the oils. Add the chives and parsley, and season with salt and pepper.

For the leeks: Wash and trim the leeks. Place them in a pan, cover with water, and bring to a boil over high heat. Reduce heat, cover, and simmer for 10 minutes or until cooked through.

Drain and cut the leeks in half lengthwise. Mix the leeks with the vinaigrette and let cool. Refrigerate and serve cold.

5.28 TOMATO AND BASIL SALAD

Ingredients

6 to 8 fresh basil leaves

6 large tomatoes (about 2 pounds)

1 shallot, minced

1 large garlic clove, minced

2 tablespoons balsamic vinegar (preferably aged)

3 tablespoons olive oil

1 tablespoon flaxseed oil (or olive oil, if flaxseed oil unavailable)

1 tablespoon minced fresh parsley

Salt

Cooking Instructions

Mince half the basil leaves and shred the remaining half.

Cut off each end of the tomatoes and discard. Slice the tomatoes and spread them on a plate. Sprinkle them with a little salt and set aside for 20 minutes.

In a bowl, mix the shallot, garlic, vinegar, and whisk in the oils. Add the minced basil and parsley, and season with salt and pepper.

Transfer the tomatoes to serving platter. Sprinkle the shredded basil, pour over the dressing, and serve immediately.

5.29 BLACK BEAN SOUP

Ingredients

12 ounces dried black beans, rinsed

2 teaspoons canola oil

1 large onion, finely diced (about 8 ounces)

2 large celery stalks, finely diced (about 4 ounces)

1 large carrot, finely diced (about 4 ounces)

2 garlic cloves, minced

6 cups chicken stock or vegetable stock (low-fat and low-sodium)

1 bouquet garni

Salt and pepper to taste

Cooking Instructions

Place the beans in a large pot and cover with water (water should go at least 2 inches above the surface of the beans). Bring to a boil over high heat. Remove from heat and let soak 1 hour. Drain and set aside.

Heat the oil in a large pan over high heat. Add the onion and sauté until translucent. Add the celery, carrot, and garlic, and cook for 2 minutes. Add the beans, stock, and bouquet garni, and bring to a boil.

Reduce heat, cover, and simmer for 45 minutes or until beans are tender. Skim off any foam forming at the liquid's surface. Remove 1/3 cup of the bean and mash with a fork. Mix the puree back into the soup. Remove the bouquet garni and season with salt and pepper. If the soup is too thick, adjust with stock. If the soup is too thin, reduce the liquid some more. Serve immediately.

5.30 CHICKPEA, TOMATO, AND RICE SOUP

Ingredients

1 teaspoon olive oil

1 small onion, diced (about 4 ounces)

3 garlic cloves, minced

1 (8 ounce) can chopped Italian plum tomatoes

1/2 teaspoon freshly minced rosemary

1/2 cup brown rice

5 cups gluten-free chicken or vegetable stock (low-fat and low-sodium)

12 ounces cooked chickpeas

2 tablespoons freshly minced parsley

Salt and pepper to taste

Cooking Instructions

Heat the oil in a large pan over high heat. Add the onion and sauté until translucent. Add the garlic, tomatoes, and rosemary, and cook until the juices are evaporated. Add the rice and stock, and bring to boil. Reduce heat, cover, and simmer for 25 minutes. Add the chickpeas and continue to cook for 5 minutes or until the rice is cooked through. Add the parsley, season with salt and pepper, and serve immediately.

5.31 GAZPACHO

Ingredients

2 slices white bread

¼ cup olive oil

3½ large tomatoes, chopped (about 1¼ pounds)

1 medium cucumber, chopped (about 8 ounces)

1 small onion, chopped (about 4 ounces)

1 small red or orange bell pepper, seeded, ribs removed, and chopped (about 3 ounces)

3 garlic cloves, chopped

1 cup tomato juice

2 tablespoons red wine vinegar

2 tablespoons chopped fresh basil

1 tablespoon freshly chopped tarragon

Dash ground cumin

Dash Tabasco sauce

½ lemon, juiced

Cayenne pepper

Salt to taste

Cooking Instructions

Soak the bread by submerging it in cold water for 5 minutes. In a blender, puree the ingredients, except salt and cayenne pepper until smooth. Add salt and cayenne pepper. Refrigerate until cold, then serve.

5.32 Lentil Soup

Ingredients

2 teaspoons canola oil

1 large onion, finely diced (about 8 ounces)

1 large carrot, finely diced (about 4 ounces)

2 large celery stalks, finely diced (about 4 ounces)

2 garlic cloves, minced

6 cups chicken stock (low-fat and low-sodium)

1 small ham bone (optional)

3 cups lentils, rinsed (about 12 ounces)

1 bouquet garni

Salt and pepper to taste

Cooking Instructions

Heat the oil in a large pan over high heat. Add the onion and sauté until translucent. Add the carrot, celery, and garlic, and cook for 2 minutes. Add the stock, ham bone, if using, lentils, and bouquet garni, and bring to a boil. Reduce heat, cover, and simmer for 35 minutes. Skim the surface to remove foam as needed. Continue to simmer uncovered for 10 minutes to thicken the soup. Remove any fat that may rise to the surface of the soup. Remove the ham bone and bouquet garni. Season with salt and pepper, and serve immediately.

5.33 ONION SOUP

Ingredients

2 tablespoons grapeseed oil

3 large onions, thinly sliced (about 1½ pounds)

2 tablespoons Cognac (optional)

2 tablespoons flour

6 to 7 cups beef stock (low-fat and low-sodium)

Salt and pepper to taste

Cooking Instructions

Heat the oil in a large pan over medium heat. Add the onions and cook until golden brown. Stir occasionally to avoid burning. This will take up to 20 minutes. Carefully add the Cognac, if using, and flambé. When the flame dies, sprinkle the flour and mix well. Add the beef stock and bring to a boil over high heat. Reduce heat and simmer for 20 to 25 minutes. Skim any foam or fat that forms. Season with salt and pepper and serve immediately.

5.34 Broiled Salmon with Dill

Ingredients

4 (5 ounce) salmon fillets

1 tablespoon olive oil

4 to 5 fresh dill branches, minced

Salt and pepper to taste

Cooking Instructions

Preheat the broiler. Rub some of the oil over the flesh side of the fillets. Lightly season with salt and pepper and spread the dill over. Place the fillets on a greased baking pan skin side up. Brush the remaining oil over the skin and broil for 3 to 4 minutes. Turn over and continue to broil for a few minutes or until the flesh starts to flake.

5.35 BROILED SALMON WITH ORANGE SALSA

Ingredients

1½ tablespoons grapeseed oil

4 (5 ounce) salmon fillets

2 mangos, diced (about 14 ounces)

1 orange, diced (about 6 ounces)

1 small red onion, diced (about 2 ounces)

2 green jalapeños, diced

1 bunch cilantro, chopped

¼ cup orange juice

Salt and pepper to taste

Cooking Instructions

Mix the mangos, orange, red onion, jalapenos, cilantro and orange juice in a bowl. Season to taste and refrigerate at least 30 minutes before use. Preheat the broiler. Brush oil over the fillets and season lightly. Broil the fish for 5 minutes on the non-skin side first. Turnover, brush more oil, and continue to cook for 5 minutes or until the flesh starts to flake. Serve immediately with the salsa.

5.36 HONEY GLAZED SALMON

Ingredients

4 (5 ounce) salmon fillets

2 tablespoons Dijon mustard

4 teaspoons honey

2 teaspoons freshly minced thyme

1 lime, Salt and pepper to taste

Cooking Instructions

Place the salmon fillets in a microwave safe dish.

In a bowl, mix the mustard, honey, thyme, and season to taste. Spread the mixture evenly over the salmon fillets. Sprinkle with a little lime juice and cover with a microwaveable top or loosely with plastic wrap. Microwave on high for 3 to 4 minutes. Time may vary based on the thickness of your fillets. Remove from the microwave and let stand for 2 minutes before serving.

5.37 BROILED TUNA WITH TARRAGON SAUCE

Ingredients

1 tablespoon olive oil

1 small shallot, minced

1 garlic clove, minced (optional)

½ cup white wine (Sauvignon Blanc)

¾ cup gluten-free vegetable stock (low-fat and low-sodium)

8 fresh tarragon branches, (4 branches minced, 4 whole)

2 tablespoons Dijon mustard

1 tablespoon cornstarch, mixed with a little water

4 (5 ounce) tuna fillets

Oil spray

2 tablespoons cream (optional)

Salt and pepper to taste

Cooking Instructions

Preheat the broiler. Heat the oil in a pan over high heat. Add the shallot and garlic, and sauté for 1 minute. Add the wine, stock, and half of the minced tarragon, and boil for 3 minutes. Strain and return liquid to the pan, discarding solids. Add the mustard and mix briefly. Add the cornstarch mixture, a little at a time, until the desired consistency is obtained. Remove from heat and set aside.

Place the fillets on a greased cookie sheet. Rub the whole tarragon branches on both sides of the fillets. Spray a little oil over the fillets and lightly season with pepper.

Broil for 4 to 5 minutes. Turn over and spray with a little more oil. Continue to broil until the flesh starts to flake. Remove the fillets and keep warm on a plate covered with aluminum foil. Reheat the prepared sauce, add the cream, if using, and the remaining minced tarragon, and bring to a boil. Season with salt and pepper and pour over the fillets. Serve immediately.

5.38 QUICK TUNA DAUBE

Ingredients

For the marinade:

3 ounces olive oil

1 lemon, juiced Pinch pepper

For the fish:

4 (5 ounce) tuna fillets

4 small canned anchovy fillets, drained and patted dry

½ cup wild rice

4 large tomatoes

1 teaspoon olive oil

1 large onion, diced (about 8 ounces)

3 garlic cloves (optional)

1 bouquet garni

1 cup Chardonnay (or other wine with citrus and butter tones)

Salt and pepper to taste

Cooking Instructions

For the marinade: Mix the oil, lemon juice, and pepper in a bowl.

For the fish: Make two small incisions in the top and bottom of each tuna fillet. Place one anchovy fillet in each incision. Place the tuna fillets in a plastic bag. Add the marinade and seal. Mix carefully and refrigerate for at least one hour.

Meanwhile, cook the rice according to package instructions. Make a small X incision at the top and bottom of the tomatoes. Blanch the tomatoes for 20 seconds. Remove and place in ice-cold water to stop the cooking process. Peel, seed, and dice the tomatoes. Set aside. Preheat the oven to 350°F. Remove the fish from the bag and pat dry with paper towels. Heat the oil in a nonstick pan over high heat. Add the tuna the pan, and brown for two to three minutes. Turn over and sauté for two minutes more. Remove the fillets from the pan and place on a platter. Cover with aluminum foil to keep warm. Deglaze the pan with a bit of water (see this page for tips on deglazing). If you prefer a less fishy smell to your dish, once deglazed disregard liquid. Add the onions and brown slightly. Add the tomatoes, garlic, bouquet garni, and wine, and bring to a boil. Transfer half of the prepared vegetables mixture to a greased casserole. Add the fish and top with the remaining vegetables mixture. Cover and bake for 20 to 25 minutes.

Remove the fish and place on a serving platter. Cover with aluminum foil to keep warm. Remove the bouquet garni. Thicken the sauce by simmering over medium heat. Season with salt and pepper and pour over the tuna fillets. Serve immediately with the wild rice.

5.39 TUNA WITH BALSAMIC VINEGAR

Ingredients

For the fish:

1 cup pearl onions

2 tablespoons olive oil

1½ cups balsamic vinegar

1 shallot, minced

1 large garlic clove, minced (optional)

1 tablespoon honey

4 (5 ounce) tuna fillets

2 tablespoons minced fresh parsley

Salt and pepper to taste

Cooking Instructions

Preheat the broiler.

Blanch the onions in boiling water for 2 minutes.

Drain, cool, and peel.

Heat 1 tablespoon of the oil in a skillet over medium heat. Add the onions and brown for two to three minutes. Add the vinegar, shallot, garlic, and honey, and reduce by half.

Meanwhile, place the fillets on a greased baking pan. Brush a little of the remaining oil over the fish and lightly season with salt and pepper. Broil for 3 to 4 minutes. Turn over, drizzle the remaining oil, and continue to cook for a few minutes or until the flesh starts to flake.

Transfer the fish to a serving platter and top with the prepared onions.

5.40 TROUT GREEK STYLE

ingredients

¼ teaspoon dried thyme

¼ teaspoon dried coriander

¼ teaspoon dried marjoram

¼ teaspoon dried rosemary

¼ teaspoon dried basil

4 (5 ounce) whole trout

1 tablespoon olive oil

4 teaspoons minced fresh parsley

4 teaspoons minced fresh mint

1 lemon, juiced

Salt and pepper to taste

Cooking Instructions

Preheat the broiler.

For the fish: In a bowl blend the dried herbs. Place the trout on a flat surface and open their cavities. Sprinkle some salt, pepper, and a large pinch of the dried herbs in each trout. Add 1 teaspoon fresh parsley and 1 teaspoon fresh mint. Sprinkle lemon juice and close the trout. Place the trout on a greased baking pan. Drizzle the oil over the trout. Broil for 3 to 4 minutes. Carefully turn over, brush with oil, and continue to broil for another 3 to 4 minutes.

5.41 TROUT WITH HORSERADISH

Ingredients

4 (5 ounce) whole trout

1 tablespoon olive oil

3 tablespoons minced fresh parsley

4 tablespoons prepared horseradish sauce (store bought)

Salt and pepper to taste

Cooking Instructions

Preheat the broiler.

Clean the fish and pat dry. Sprinkle the inside of each trout with a little salt, pepper, oil, and parsley. Place the trout on a greased baking pan. Rub a little oil over the skin. Broil for 3 to 4 minutes. Carefully turn over, brush with oil, and continue to broil for another 3 to 4 minutes. Serve immediately with the prepared horseradish sauce.

5.42 MACKEREL WITH STEAMED VEGETABLES

Ingredients

For the fish:

4 (5 ounce) mackerels

1 large garlic clove, peeled

2 tablespoons olive oil

Salt and pepper

For the vegetables:

4 large carrots, sliced (about 1 pound)

3 large zucchini, sliced (about 1 pound)

1 lemon, quartered

Salt and pepper to taste

Cooking Instructions

For the fish: Pre-heat the oven to 400°F. Sprinkle pepper and a little salt inside the mackerels. Cut the garlic clove in half and brush each half all over the bottom of a baking pan. Sprinkle half of the oil over the bottom of the pan and add the mackerel. Spread the remaining oil over the fish and bake for 20 to 25 minutes.

For the vegetables: Preheat a steamer. Add the carrots and cook for 4 minutes. Add the zucchini and continue to cook for 2 to 3 minutes or until desired tenderness. Transfer to a serving platter and season to taste. Serve the mackerels with the vegetables and lemon wedges.

5.43 ITALIAN-STYLE MONKFISH

Ingredients

6 large tomatoes (about 2 pounds)

½ cup brown rice

1 tablespoon olive oil

4 (5 ounce) monkfish fillets

1 large onion, sliced (about 8 ounces)

2 tablespoons minced garlic (optional)

1 large green bell pepper, seeded, ribs removed, and sliced (about 8 ounces)

1 large yellow bell pepper, seeded, ribs removed, and sliced (about 8 ounces)

2 pinches Italian herbs

1 bunch fresh basil, shredded

Salt and pepper to taste

Cooking Instructions

Make a small X incision at the top and bottom of the tomatoes. Blanch the tomatoes for 20 seconds. Remove and place in ice-cold water to stop the cooking process. Peel, seed, and slice the tomatoes. Cook the rice according to package instructions. Heat the oil in a large nonstick pan over high heat. Lightly season the fish with salt and pepper, add to the pan, and brown for two to three minutes. Turn over and sauté for 2 minutes more. Remove the fish and set aside on a plate. Deglaze the pan with a little water (see above for tips on deglazing). Add the onions and cook for 2 minutes. Add the garlic, tomatoes, bell peppers, and Italian herbs, and sauté for 2 minutes. Slide the fillets back into the pan, cover, and cook for 20 minutes over low heat. Remove the fillets and place on a serving platter. Cover with aluminum foil to keep warm. Mix the basil into the vegetables and season with salt and pepper. Pour over the fish and serve immediately with the rice.

Scallops With Tangerines

Ingredients

6 tangerines

1 cup orange juice

1 teaspoon minced ginger

3 teaspoons olive oil, plus more for drizzling

1 pound scallops

1 shallot, minced

8 ounces mushrooms

2 tablespoons minced fresh parsley

Salt and pepper

Cooking Instructions

Peel and segment the tangerines. Place the orange juice and half of the ginger in a saucepan and bring to a boil over high heat. Reduce to ¼ cup and set aside.

Heat 1 teaspoon oil in a saucepan over high heat. Add the mushrooms, shallot, and remaining ginger, and sauté briefly. Add parsley and lightly season with salt and pepper. Heat the remaining 2 teaspoons oil in a large saucepan over high heat. Lightly season the scallops, add to the pan, and sear for 1½ minutes. Turn over and sear for 1½ minutes more. Add the tangerine segments, reduced orange juice, and continue to sauté for 1 minute. Serve immediately with the mushrooms and drizzle a little oil.

5.44 SEA BASS WITH GINGER AND LIME

Ingredients

For the fish:

1 tablespoon olive oil

4 (5 ounce) sea bass fillets

½ cup lime juice

½ small onion, diced (about 2 ounces)

1 teaspoon minced garlic (optional)

1 tablespoon minced fresh ginger

½ cup Chardonnay wine (or other wine with lemon-lime tones)

1 tablespoon honey

1 teaspoon fresh rosemary Cornstarch mixed with a
little water

2 tablespoons minced fresh parsley

Salt and pepper to taste

For the vegetables:

1 pound carrots

1 pound green beans

1 lime, juiced

Salt and pepper to taste

Cooking Instructions

For the vegetables: Steam vegetables until desired tenderness. Mix with lemon juice, season with sea salt and pepper, and set aside.

For the fish: Heat the oil in a nonstick pan over medium heat. Lightly season the fillets with salt and pepper, add to the pan, and brown for two to three minutes. Turn over and cook for 2 minutes more.

Add about ⅓ of the lime juice, cover, and reduce heat. Cook the fillets until the flesh starts to flake. Remove the fish from the pan and place on a serving platter. Cover with aluminum foil to keep warm. Add the onions, garlic, ginger, wine, remaining lime juice, honey, and rosemary to the pan. Mix well and bring to a boil. Reduce the sauce to ⅔ cup. Add a little of the cornstarch mixture and bring to a boil to thicken. Strain, discarding solids, and return to pan. Add the parsley and adjust seasoning. Pour over the fillets and serve immediately with the cooked vegetables.

5.45 SHRIMP SCAMPI

Ingredients

For the pasta:

½ cup whole wheat pasta

For the shrimp:

4 tablespoons olive oil

2 garlic cloves, minced (optional)

2 pounds large shrimp, shelled and deveined

2 red bell peppers, seeded, ribs removed, and sliced (about 1 pound)

½ lemon, zest removed and juiced

2 tablespoons minced fresh parsley

Salt and pepper to taste

Cooking Instructions

For the pasta: Cook according to package directions.

For the shrimp: Heat the oil and garlic in a large pan over medium heat. Add the shrimp and cook for 1 minute stirring occasionally. Add the bell peppers, lemon zest and juice, parsley, and season with salt and pepper. Continue to cook for two minutes or until the shrimp is cooked through stirring occasionally. Add the cooked pasta, toss, and serve immediately.

5.46 CHICKEN BREAST WITH DIJON MUSTARD

Ingredients

4 (5 ounce) skinless chicken breasts Canola oil

1 tablespoon Dijon mustard

2 teaspoons lemon juice

½ teaspoon garlic powder (optional)

Salt and pepper to taste

Cooking Instructions

Preheat the oven to 375°F. Place the chicken breasts in a lightly oiled pan. In a bowl, mix the mustard, lemon juice, and garlic powder. Spread over the chicken breasts and season to taste. Bake for 20 to 25 minutes, or until cooked through. Time may vary depending on the thickness of the breasts.

Ingredients

4 teaspoons olive oil

4 tablespoons dried Italian herbs

4 (6 ounce) bone-in, skin-on chicken breasts

1 large lemon, cut in 8 slices

Pepper to taste

Cooking Instructions

Preheat the oven to 375°F. Mix the olive oil, Italian herbs, and season with pepper. With your fingers, carefully separate the chicken skin slightly from the flesh, being careful not to break the skin. Spread the herbed oil mixture over the chicken flesh, add 2 lemon slices per breast, and push back the skin. Place the breasts in a baking dish and bake for 20 to 25 minutes, or until cooked through. Time may vary depending on the thickness of the breasts. Serve immediately and remember to discard the skin when eating.

5.48 ROASTED CHICKEN BREAST WITH SWEET POTATOES

Ingredients

2 tablespoons olive oil

4 (4 ounce) skinless chicken breasts

4 sweet potatoes, unpeeled and quartered (about 1 pound)

1 large yellow bell pepper, seeded, ribs removed, and chopped (about 8 ounces)

1 large zucchini, chopped (about 8 ounces)

1 teaspoon dried Italian herbs

Salt and pepper to taste

Cooking Instructions

Preheat the oven to 400°F.

In large bowl mix 1 tablespoon oil with the chicken and transfer to a roasting pan. Toss the remaining 1 tablespoon oil with the sweet potatoes, bell pepper, and zucchini. Transfer to the roasting pan arranging them around the chicken breasts. Sprinkle the Italian herbs and lightly season with pepper. Roast until the chicken and vegetables are tender, 25 to 30 minutes, turning halfway through the cooking time. Remove from the oven, season lightly with salt, and serve immediately.

5.49 CHICKEN BURGERS WITH LETTUCE WRAPS

Ingredients

2 white anchovy fillets

4 tablespoons garlic Caesar Litehouse Foods dressing

4 (4 ounce) organic chicken burgers

2 tablespoons olive oil

4 garlic cloves, minced (optional)

16 lettuce leaves

4 tablespoons Parmesan cheese

Canola oil

Salt and pepper to taste

Cooking Instructions

In a food processor, puree the anchovy fillets with the dressing. Add a little water to thin out. Lightly season the burgers with salt and pepper and shape them to fit in the lettuce leaves. Do not allow the meat to touch the leaves. Heat up the olive oil with the garlic. Remove at first boil and set aside.

Preheat the grill to medium-high heat. Grease the grill with canola oil before adding the burgers. Cook them for 3 to 5 minutes on each side or until cooked through. Meanwhile, carefully brush the garlic oil over the lettuce leaves.

Place two leaves on a plate, top with one burger, spread 1 tablespoon of the dressing, sprinkle 1 tablespoon cheese, and fold any lettuce overhang over the top. Top with 2 more leaves and tuck underneath to seal. Repeat with the remaining ingredients. Serve immediately with your favorite sides. Use toothpick to hold the lettuce in place if necessary

5.50 NEW YORK STEAK WITH MUSHROOMS AND ONIONS

Ingredients

4 (4 ounce) New York steaks

5 teaspoons olive oil

1 pound onions, sliced (about 2 large onions)

1 pound mushrooms, sliced

2 garlic cloves, minced (optional)

2 tablespoons freshly minced parsley

¼ cup Dijon mustard

Salt and pepper to taste

Cooking Instructions

Preheat the broiler. Brush 1 teaspoon each of the olive oil over the steaks and season with pepper. Broil for 3 to 5 minutes on each side or to desired tenderness. Sprinkle a little salt before serving.

Meanwhile, heat the remaining 1 teaspoon olive oil in a nonstick pan over medium heat. Add the onions and brown slightly. Add the mushrooms and garlic, and continue to cook until the mushrooms are slightly tender. Add the parsley and season with salt and pepper.

Plate the vegetables in the center of a serving platter and top with the steaks. Serve with Dijon mustard on the side.

5.51   CORNISH HEN WITH RED CABBAGE

Ingredients

2 tablespoons grapeseed oil

2 Cornish hens

4 slices turkey bacon

1 large onion, sliced (about 8 ounces)

2 Granny Smith apple, sliced (about 8 ounces)

1 red cabbage, sliced (about 1½ pounds)

4 cups chicken stock (low-fat and low-sodium)

2 cloves

1 laurel leaf

1 teaspoon caraway seeds

Mustard

Salt and pepper to taste

Cooking Instructions

Blanch the red cabbage into boiling salted water. Rinse the Cornish hen under cold water, pat dry, and lightly season.

Heat half of the oil in a sauté pan. Sear the Cornish hen on all sides (about 10 minutes).

Heat the remaining oil in a Dutch oven or brasier. Add the bacon, onion, apples, and sweat for two minutes. Add the red cabbage, stock, cloves, laurel leaf, caraway seeds, and bring to boil. Top with the Cornish hen, cover, and cook for 40 to 50 minutes in the oven. Serve with mustard on the side.

5.52 LAMB CHOPS WITH HERBS

Ingredients

1 tablespoon minced garlic (optional)

1 tablespoon minced fresh parsley

4 tablespoons whole wheat bread crumbs

1 tablespoon minced fresh Italian herbs

3 tablespoons Dijon mustard Olive oil

8 (3½ ounce) lamb loin chops (about 1¾ pounds total)

Salt and pepper to taste

Cooking Instructions

Preheat the oven to 400°F.

In a bowl, combine the garlic, parsley, bread crumbs, and Italian herbs, then season with salt and pepper. Add the mustard and just enough oil to bind the mixture together.

Heat 1 teaspoon oil in a sauté pan over high heat. Add the lamb chops and brown on both sides, about three to four minutes each side. Remove from heat. Place the chops on a greased baking pan. Spread the breadcrumb mixture over the chops and press hard. Bake for 10 minutes for medium rare or up to 15 minutes for welldone.

5.53 MEATLOAF WITH TOMATO SAUCE

Ingredients

1 teaspoon olive oil

1 small onion, minced (about 4 ounces)

1 celery stalk, minced (about 2 ounces)

2 garlic cloves, minced (optional)

1 pound ground buffalo meat

¾ pound ground chicken or turkey meat

3 ounces gluten-free ground oats

1 large egg, beaten

3 ounces chicken stock (low-fat and low-sodium)

1 teaspoon salt

¼ teaspoon pepper

½ teaspoon dried Italian herbs

¼ teaspoon dry mustard

⅛ teaspoon dried sage

10 ounces diced tomato

1 cup tomato sauce

Cooking Instructions

Preheat the oven to 350°F.

Heat the oil in a pan over high heat. Add the onion, celery, and garlic, and cook for 2 minutes. Transfer to a mixing bowl and add the remaining ingredients, except the tomato sauce. Mix well and place the meat-loaf into a greased loaf pan. Bake for 1 hour to 1½ hours or until cooked through. Serve with your favorite tomato sauce.

5.54 TURKEY BREAST WITH SAGE AROMAS

Ingredients

2 tablespoons olive oil

1 turkey breast (about 2 pounds)

1 tablespoon ground sage

3 to 4 fresh sage leaves

½ cup chicken stock (low-fat and low-sodium)

Cornstarch

Salt and pepper to taste

Cooking Instructions

Preheat the oven to 350°F.

Mix the ground sage with a little pepper and spread all over the turkey breast under its skin. Be careful not to break the skin. Brush olive oil over the skin. Place the turkey skin-side up in a roasting pan. Pour the chicken stock in the pan, add the sage leaves, and bake for an hour or until a meat thermometer registers 180°F.

Remove the turkey breast from the pan, cover with aluminum foil to keep warm. Remove the sage leaves from the sauce and thicken with a little cornstarch and water mixture. Adjust seasonings and serve over the turkey breast slices.

5.55 MEDITERRANEAN PORTOBELLO BURGER

Ingredients

4 teaspoons olive oil

4 large portobello mushroom caps

4 slices onion

2 garlic cloves, minced (optional)

4 tablespoons roasted red bell pepper spread

4 teaspoons chopped black olives

4 teaspoons feta cheese

8 slices tomato

8 large basil leaves

Lettuce leaves wide enough to wrap portobello mushrooms

Apple cider vinegar

Pepper to taste

Cooking Instructions

Preheat the grill to medium heat.

Brush 1 teaspoon olive oil and sprinkle pepper over each portobello. Grill the mushrooms for 2 minutes on each side. Add the onion and grill. Turn the mushrooms so that the top of the mushroom cap is on the grill. Fill the underside cavity with the garlic, bell pepper spread, and olives, and season with salt and pepper. Grill for another minute or two.

Place each portobello mushroom on a few lettuce leaves (cap side down), add 1 teaspoon feta cheese, 1 grilled onion slice, 2 slices tomato, 2 basil leaves, and sprinkle vinegar. Close the lettuce leaves to seal and serve immediately.

5.56 CHICKEN BREAST WITH ASIAN GLAZE

Ingredients

4 (5 ounce) chicken breasts with bones and skin

2 tablespoons maple syrup

1 tablespoon green tea leaves

1 tablespoon Oriental hot mustard

1 garlic clove, minced

2 tablespoons sesame seeds

1 teaspoon ground ginger

Canola oil

Salt and pepper to taste

Cooking Instructions

Preheat the oven to 350°F. Wash and pat dry the chicken breasts. Carefully pass your fingers between the meat and the skin to loosen up the skin without breaking it.

Heat the maple syrup, tea, mustard, garlic, and ginger in a saucepan over low heat until well blended. Season to taste and set aside. Lift up the chicken skin and brush the mixture over the chicken meat. Sprinkle the sesame seeds under the skin. Brush canola oil over the skin and roast for 30 minutes, or until cooked through. Remove skin before serving.

5.57 CHICKEN BREAST WITH WILD MUSHROOMS

Ingredients

2 teaspoons olive oil

4 (5 ounce) skinless chicken breasts

2 shallots, minced

3 garlic cloves, minced

½ cup red wine (Syrah, Shiraz, or Barbaresco)

1 cup chicken stock (low-fat and low-sodium)

2 fresh rosemary sprigs

Cornstarch mixed with a little water

1 tablespoon minced fresh parsley

Salt and pepper to taste

For the side:

2 teaspoons olive oil

1 pound wild mushrooms, cleaned and sliced

1 pound cooked chestnuts

1 tablespoon minced fresh parsley

Salt and pepper to taste

Cooking Instructions

For the chicken: Heat the oil in a sauté pan over high heat. Lightly season the chicken with salt and pepper, add to the pan, and brown on both sides for three minutes each side. Add the shallots, garlic, wine, and reduce by half. Add ½ cup of the chicken stock and 2 sprigs rosemary, and bring to a boil. Reduce heat, cover, and simmer for 10 to 15 minutes or until the chicken is cooked through.

Remove the chicken breasts from the pan and place on a serving platter. Cover with aluminum foil to keep warm. Add the remaining ½ cup stop stock to the pan and reduce the liquids to a little less than 1 cup. Thicken with a little cornstarch mixture. Add the parsley together with, any rendered chicken juices, and bring to a boil. Adjust seasonings and pour over the chicken.

For the side: Heat oil in a nonstick pan over medium heat. Add the mushrooms and cook until almost cooked through. Add the chestnuts, mix well, season to taste, and continue to cook for 2 to 3 minutes. Add a little sauce from the chicken and mix well.

Serve the chicken breasts with the mushrooms and chestnuts.

5.58 LEMON CHICKEN

Ingredients

3 tablespoons olive oil

5 lemons (4 juiced, 1 cut into wedges)

1 tablespoon freshly minced poultry herbs

4 (4 ounce) skinless chicken breasts

Pepper to taste

Cooking Instructions

Mix in 2 tablespoons of the oil, the juice, and herbs, and season with pepper. Place the chicken pieces in a plastic bag. Pour the lemon marinade over the chicken and refrigerate for at least one hour rotating every 10 minutes.

Preheat the broiler. Remove the chicken breasts from the marinade and pat dry. Place them on a cookie sheet greased with a little of the remaining 1 tablespoon oil and brush the rest of the remaining oil over each breast. Broil for approximately 6 to 7 minutes on each side. Watch carefully to avoid burning. Serve immediately with the lemon wedges.

5.59 STUFFED CHICKEN BREAST WITH BOURSIN

Ingredients

4 (4 ounce) chicken breasts

4 pinches dried Italian herbs

2 ounces Boursin (garlic and herbs), divided into four portions

8 fresh large basil leaves

1 tablespoon olive oil, plus more for stir-frying

1 large shallot, thinly sliced

1 cup chicken stock (low-fat and low-sodium)

Cornstarch mixed with a little water

2 tablespoons minced fresh parsley

2 pounds fresh dandelions, washed and pat dry

Salt and pepper to taste

Kitchen twine or toothpicks

Cooking Instructions

Preheat the oven to 350°F. Place the chicken breasts between two plastic wrap sheets. Flatten with a mallet until fairly thin. Sprinkle pepper and a pinch of Italian herbs on each breast. Spread one portion of Boursin and 2 basil leaves, and roll each breast tightly. Secure with kitchen twine so they do not unroll. Heat the oil in an ovenproof sauté pan over high heat. Add the turkey rolls, side face down, and brown for two to three minutes. Turn over and brown two minutes more. Once browned, add the shallot and ½ cup of the chicken stock. Bring to a boil and place in the oven for 10 to 12 minutes. Remove the rolls from the pan and place on a serving platter. Cover with aluminum foil to keep warm. Add the remaining ½ cup stock to the pan (be careful, it just came out of the oven!) and reduce the sauce to a little less than 1 cup. Thicken with a little cornstarch mixture. Add the parsley and any rendered turkey juices, and bring to a boil. Adjust seasonings and pour over the turkey. Serve immediately with the steamed dandelions. While the sauce is reducing, stir-fry the dandelions until slightly wilted. Season to taste and serve with the stuffed chicken.

5.60 LAMB CHOPS WITH GARLIC SPREAD

Ingredients

4 cups green beans (about 2 pounds)

6 teaspoons olive oil

2 tablespoons minced garlic

2 teaspoons freshly minced parsley

2 teaspoons freshly minced rosemary

½ teaspoon dry crushed red pepper

4 (4 ounce) loin lamb chops

Salt and pepper to taste

Cooking Instructions

Trim and place the green beans in a pan. Cover with water, add 1 teaspoon of salt, and bring to boil. Reduce heat and simmer until tender. Drain and transfer to a serving bowl. Add 2 teaspoons olive oil, season with salt and pepper, and mix well.

In a bowl, mix 2 teaspoons of the remaining oil, the garlic, parsley, rosemary, and dry crushed red pepper. Rub the spread over the lamb chops.

Heat the remaining 2 teaspoons oil in a nonstick pan over medium heat. Add the lamb chops and cook for 3 to 4 minutes on each side or to desired doneness. Serve immediately with the prepared green beans.

5.61 Pork Loin with Tomato Coulis

Ingredients

6 large tomatoes (about 2 pounds)

1 tablespoon olive oil

4 (5 ounce) pork loin chops

3 garlic cloves, minced

2 shallots, minced

Pinch sugar

1 tablespoon flour

½ cup Chardonnay

½ cup vegetable stock (low-fat and low-sodium)

1 teaspoon tomato paste

1 fresh rosemary sprig

Cornstarch mixed with a little water

2 tablespoons minced fresh basil

2 tablespoons minced fresh parsley

Salt and pepper to taste

Cooking Instructions

Make a small X incision on the top and bottom of the tomatoes. Blanch the tomatoes for 20 seconds. Place in ice-cold water to stop the cooking process. Peel, seed, and dice the tomatoes.

Heat the oil in a deep pan over high heat. Lightly season the loin chops with salt and pepper, add to the pan, and brown on both sides, about three to four minutes each side. Add the garlic, shallots, diced tomatoes, and sugar, and reduce heat to medium. Sprinkle the flour over the vegetables and mix well. Continue to cook for 2 minutes. Add the wine, stock, tomato paste, and rosemary, and bring to a boil. Cover and cook for 25 minutes over low heat.

Remove the chops and set aside in a serving platter. Cover with aluminum foil to keep warm. Remove the rosemary and puree the sauce with a hand mixer or in a blender. Reduce the sauce to concentrate its flavors. If necessary, thicken with a little cornstarch mixture. Add the basil, parsley, any rendered loins juices, and bring to a boil. Adjust seasonings and pour over the chops.

5.62 STUFFED TURKEY BREAST ITALIAN STYLE

Ingredients

4 (4 ounce) skinless turkey breasts

4 pinches dried Italian herbs

4 slices prosciutto ham

2 ounces goat cheese, sliced in 4 pieces

8 large fresh basil leaves

1 tablespoon olive oil

1 large shallot, thinly sliced ¼ cup Madeira

1 cup chicken stock (low-fat and low-sodium)

Cornstarch mixed with a little water

2 tablespoons minced fresh parsley

Salt and pepper to taste

Toothpicks or kitchen twine

Cooking Instructions

Preheat the oven to 350°F.

Place the turkey breasts between two plastic wrap sheets. Flatten with a mallet until fairly thin. Lightly season with salt and pepper, and sprinkle a pinch of Italian herbs on each breast. To each breast add one slice of ham, one slice of cheese, and 2 basil leaves, and roll tightly. Secure with a few toothpicks so they do not unroll.

Heat the oil in an ovenproof sauté pan over high heat. Add the turkey rolls, folded side down, and brown, about two to three minutes. Turn over and sauté, two minutes more. Once browned, add the shallot, Madeira, ½ cup of the chicken stock. Bring to a boil and place in the oven for 10 to 12 minutes. Remove the rolls from the oven and place on a serving platter. Cover with aluminum foil to keep warm. Add the remaining ½ cup stock to the pan (be careful, it just came out of the oven!) and reduce the sauce to with a little less than 1 cup. Thicken with a little cornstarch mixture. Add the parsley and any rendered turkey juices, and bring to a boil. Adjust seasonings and pour over the turkey.

5.63 Turkey Breast with Cherries

Ingredients

½ cup brown rice

1 tablespoon grapeseed oil

4 turkey breasts

1 large shallot, minced

1 teaspoon black peppercorns, cracked

2 pinches dried thyme

1 bay leaf

1 cinnamon stick

1 cup pomegranate juice

1 cup brown sauce

1 cup pitted cherries

2 tablespoons minced fresh parsley

Salt and pepper to taste

Cooking Instructions

Preheat the oven to 350°F.

Cook the rice according to the package instructions. Heat the oil in an ovenproof skillet over high heat. Lightly season the turkey breasts with salt and pepper, add to the pan, and brown on both sides. Transfer to the oven and continue to cook for 10 minutes. Remove the pan from the oven with oven mitt and transfer the turkey breasts to a plate. Cover with aluminum foil to keep warm. Handling the pan with the oven mitt, discard any fat from the pan. Add the shallot, peppercorns, thyme, bay leaf, cinnamon, and pomegranate juice, and deglaze the bottom and sides of the pan (see this page for tips on deglazing). Bring to a boil and reduce by half. Remove the cinnamon stick. Add the brown sauce and reduce the sauce to 1 cup. Add the cherries and bring to a boil. Add the turkey breasts back to the pan with any rendered juices, and bring to a boil. Add the parsley. Bring to a simmer, adjust seasonings, and serve immediately.

5.64 Tuscan Beef Stew

Ingredients

6 teaspoons olive oil

6 ounces onion, diced (about 1 medium onion)

2 garlic cloves, minced

2 pounds lean beef stew meat

½ cup Tuscan red wine (or beef stock)

6 ounces celery stalks, sliced (about 3 celery stalks)

2 whole cloves

2½ cups diced tomatoes

3 parsley branches, minced

3 medium potatoes, quartered (about 18 ounces potatoes)

1 bouquet garni, Salt and pepper to taste

Cooking Instructions

Heat 2 teaspoons of oil in a pan over high heat. Add the onion and garlic, and sauté until translucent. Transfer to a stockpot. Using the same pan, add 2 teaspoons of the remaining oil and brown half the meat. Transfer the meat to the stockpot and repeat the process with the remaining 2 teaspoons oil and beef. Deglaze the pan with the wine (or stock), swirling to dissolve the particles on the bottom and sides of the pan. Transfer the deglazing liquid to the stockpot.

Heat the stockpot over medium heat. Add the celery, cloves, tomatoes, parsley, and bouquet garni, and season with pepper. Cook over low heat for 1 hour. Add the potatoes and continue to cook for 20 minutes. If the meat is not tender enough, remove the potatoes, and continue to cook until tender. Adjust seasonings and serve immediately.

5.65 Pasta with Vegetables and Sun-Dried Tomatoes

Ingredients

8 ounces penne

4 teaspoons olive oil

½ small onion, diced (about 2 ounces)

1 medium yellow bell pepper, diced (about 6 ounces)

2 garlic cloves, minced

Florets from 1 large head broccoli (about 8 ounces)

10 sun-dried tomatoes packed in oil, julienned, plus some of the packing oil

¼ teaspoon red pepper flakes

2 tablespoons pine nuts

1 bunch fresh basil leaves, julienned

Salt and pepper to taste

Cooking Instructions

Cook the pasta according to package directions. Drain and return to the pan. Mix in 1 teaspoon of the oil.

Heat 2 teaspoons of the oil in a pan over high heat. Add the onion and sauté until translucent. Add the bell peppers and garlic, and cook for 2 minutes, mixing occasionally. Add the broccoli and sun-dried tomatoes, and continue to cook until the vegetables are tender. Add a little of the oil from the sun-dried tomatoes, the pine nuts and basil, and season with salt and pepper. Blend in the cooked pasta and serve immediately.

5.66 Tofu and Collard Greens Burgers

Ingredients

8 ounces tofu

6 ounces cooked collard greens

1 small onion, diced (about 4 ounces)

1 small carrot, shredded (about 2 ounces)

2 scallions, chopped

2 garlic cloves, minced (optional)

1⅓ cups water crackers

4 teaspoons almond butter

2 tablespoons minced salad herbs

Salt and pepper to taste

Cooking Instructions

Mix all the ingredients in a food processor until well combined. Form 4 patties and grill on each side for 4 to 5 minutes. Serve immediately.

5.67 BABY BELL PEPPERS WITH TUNA

Ingredients

12 ounces tuna canned in water

2 tablespoons minced fresh parsley

2 tablespoons minced fresh chives

¼ cup finely chopped scallions

1 lemon, juiced

6 tablespoons canola mayonnaise

24 baby bell peppers (approximately 4 cups)

Salt and pepper to taste

Cooking Instructions

In a bowl, mix the tuna, parsley, chives, and scallions. Sprinkle a little bit of lemon juice. Mix in the mayonnaise and season with salt and pepper. Refrigerate until needed.

Cut off the tops of the bell peppers. Remove the seeds and ribs. Fill with the tuna mixture and serve immediately.

5.68 BUTTERNUT SQUASH WITH CINNAMON

Ingredients

2 pounds butternut squash

1 orange (about 6 ounces)

3 tablespoons maple syrup

1 teaspoon cinnamon

1½ tablespoons grapeseed oil

Salt and pepper to taste

Cooking Instructions

Preheat the oven to 350°F.

Remove two large zest strips from the orange. Mince and set aside. Juice the orange and set aside.

Halve the squash lengthwise and remove the seeds and strings. Rub the inside with grapeseed oil and season to taste. Place on a greased cookie sheet, skin side down, and bake for 35 to 40 minutes or until tender.

Meanwhile heat the orange juice, maple syrup, and cinnamon in a pan over high heat. Reduce by half.

Remove the squash from the oven, scoop out the flesh, and transfer to a food processor. Add the orange zest, 1 tablespoon of the concentrated juice, and purée. Add more concentrated juice as needed to reach the desired thickness. Adjust seasonings and serve immediately.

5.69 PROVENCE-STYLE TOMATOES

Ingredients

4 large tomatoes

6 teaspoons olive oil

1 bunch fresh basil leaves, minced

¼ cup wheat breadcrumbs

Salt and pepper to taste

Cooking Instructions

Preheat the oven to 375°F.

Cut the tomatoes in half. Lightly season with salt and pepper and sprinkle ¼ teaspoon oil over each tomato half. Add some basil and 1 teaspoon breadcrumbs over each half. Place in a baking dish. Sprinkle remaining oil over the breadcrumbs. Bake for 20 to 25 minutes and serve immediately.

5.70 FRENCH MACARONI AND CHEESE

Ingredients

8 ounces whole wheat macaroni

2 tablespoons unsalted butter

4 ounces Gruyère cheese, finely shredded

¼ cup 2% low-fat milk, heated

Pinch nutmeg

Salt and pepper to taste

Cooking Instructions

Cook the macaroni according to package directions. Drain and return to the pan. Over very low heat, mix in the butter, Gruyère, and milk. Continue to mix until the cheese is melted. Remove from heat and add a pinch of nutmeg. Season with salt and pepper, and serve immediately.

Gruyère cheese is what makes this dish so unique. However, if not available, you may substitute Swiss cheese.

5.71 GREEN BEANS WITH TOMATOES

Ingredients

1 pound green beans, ends trimmed

1½ tablespoons olive oil

½ cup pearl onions, peeled and halved

2 garlic cloves, minced (optional)

1 cup cherry tomatoes

2 pinches minced fresh thyme

2 tablespoons minced fresh basil

1 tablespoon minced fresh parsley

Pepper to taste

Cooking Instructions

Bring to a boil enough water to cover the green beans. Add 1 teaspoon of salt. Add the green beans and bring to a boil. Reduce heat and simmer until cooked through. Drain and set aside.

Heat 1 tablespoon of the oil in a sauté pan over medium heat. Add the pearl onions and sauté until golden brown. Add the garlic and cook for 1 minute. Add the green beans, tomatoes, and herbs, and cook until the vegetables are warmed through. Blend in the remaining oil, season with salt and pepper, and serve immediately.

5.72 STUFFED MUSHROOMS WITH TAPENADE

Ingredients

24 large mushrooms, stems removed

1 cup pitted black olives

1 ounce capers, drained, rinsed, and patted dry

2 ounces anchovy fillets

2 garlic cloves, minced (optional)

3 ounces olive oil

1 bunch fresh parsley, minced

1 teaspoon lemon juice

Cooking Instructions

Preheat the broiler. Empty and clean the center of each mushroom caps. Place the mushrooms on a baking sheet. Broil for 3 to 4 minutes until the mushrooms start to sweat. Do not overcook, as the mushrooms will start to shrink. Remove from the oven and set aside to cool.

In a food processor, puree the olives, capers, anchovies, garlic, oil, and lemon juice. Add pepper to taste. Fill each mushroom cap with the tapenade, sprinkle with parsley, and serve immediately.

5.73 SALMON BRUSCHETTA

Ingredients

1⅓ cups fresh basil

⅔ cup fresh parsley

2 tablespoons minced fresh lemon thyme

½ cup walnuts

2 garlic cloves (optional)

1 lemon, zested and juiced

¼ cup olive oil

1 country bread loaf

24 smoked salmon slices, rolled (about 1 pound, 2 ounces)

Salt and pepper to taste

Cooking Instructions

In a food processor, puree the basil, parsley, lemon thyme, walnuts, garlic, 1 tablespoon lemon zest, and 1 tablespoon lemon juice. Gradually add the oil until you have a smooth paste. Season with salt and pepper. If too thick, add a little more oil.

Preheat the broiler. With a serrated knife, cut the walnut bread into ½-inch-thick slices. Cut each slice in half. Place the slices on a baking sheet. Broil on both sides until golden brown. Cool before using.

Spread some paste over each bread slice. Add one salmon roll, sprinkle each with a little lemon juice, and serve immediately.

5.74 Sugar Snap Peas with Salmon

Ingredients

1 tablespoon olive oil

2 cups sugar snap peas

2 garlic cloves, minced (optional)

1 lemon

4 ounces salmon, thinly sliced

Salt and pepper to taste

Cooking Instructions

Remove strings along both lengths of the sugar snap peas. Heat a wok with the olive oil over medium heat. Add the garlic and sauté quickly. Add the sugar snap peas and sauté until almost tender. Add the salmon and sauté quickly. Sprinkle with lemon juice, season to taste, and serve immediately.

5.75 STUFFED EGGPLANT

Ingredients

1 egg

½ cup wheat breadcrumbs

½ teaspoon dried Italian herbs, minced

2 medium eggplants (about 1 pound)

Olive oil

1 medium onion, diced (about 6 ounces)

1 tablespoon minced garlic (optional)

4 basil leaves, minced

¼ cup minced fresh parsley

Salt and pepper to taste

Cooking Instructions

Place the egg in a saucepan and cover with water. Bring to a boil over medium heat and cook for 10 minutes. Drain and cool in cold water. Peel the egg and mash with a fork in a bowl. Meanwhile, mix the breadcrumbs and dried Italian herbs.

Preheat the oven to 425°F. Cut the eggplants in half and remove the flesh without damaging the skin. Make very small incisions on the rim tops to allow the skin to stretch a bit, this will prevent breakage during cooking. Place the eggplant halves in a small greased baking pan and brush them with oil. Set aside. In a food processor puree the eggplant flesh and mashed egg. Heat 1 teaspoon oil in a nonstick pan over medium heat. Add the onions and garlic, and sauté for 2 minutes. Add the eggplant mixture and fresh herbs, and cook for 2 minutes more. Season with salt and pepper and fill the eggplant cavities with this mixture. Sprinkle the herbed breadcrumbs over the eggplant halves and sprinkle with a little olive oil. Bake for 30 to 35 minutes.

5.76 VEGETABLES GRATIN

Ingredients

1 large yellow squash, chopped large (about 8 ounces)

1 large red bell pepper; seeded, ribs removed, and chopped large (about 8 ounces)

1 large green bell pepper; seeded, ribs removed, and chopped large (about 8 ounces)

1 large zucchini, chopped large (about 8 ounces)

1 large onion, quartered (about 8 ounces)

2 medium sweet potatoes, chopped large (about 8 ounces)

2 garlic cloves, minced (optional)

2 tablespoons lemon juice

2 tablespoons olive oil

1 fresh thyme branch, minced

2 tablespoons freshly minced parsley

2 tablespoons grated Parmesan cheese

Salt and pepper to taste

Cooking Instructions

Cut the vegetables the same size for even cooking.

In a bowl mix the garlic, lemon juice, thyme, parsley, and season to taste. Mix in the remaining vegetables (except sweet potatoes) and set aside for at least an hour.

Preheat the oven to 425°F. Place the sweet potatoes in a roasting pan. Mix in half of the olive oil, sprinkle with pepper, and bake for 20 minutes. Sprinkle the remaining oil over the potatoes. Add the prepared vegetables with the marinade and continue to bake for 20 minutes. Sprinkle the cheese, brown under the broiler, and serve immediately.

5.77 RICE WITH LENTILS

Ingredients

2½ cups lentils, rinsed

2 teaspoons olive oil

2 large onions, diced (about 1 pound)

2 teaspoons minced garlic

1 teaspoon ground cumin

1 teaspoon ground coriander

1 teaspoon paprika

2 tablespoons minced fresh parsley

1⅓ cups long-grain rice, rinsed

Salt and pepper to taste

Cooking Instructions

Place the lentils in a pan and add enough water to cover them. Bring to a boil over high heat and simmer for 10 minutes. Drain and set aside.

Heat the oil in a large pan over high heat. Add the onions and sauté until translucent. Add the garlic, lentils, cumin, coriander, paprika, and parsley, and season with salt and pepper. Add 6 cups water. Bring to a boil, reduce heat, cover, and simmer for 10 minutes. Add the rice and bring to a boil. Reduce heat, cover, and cook for 20 minutes or until tender.

Adjust seasonings and remove from heat. Set aside covered for 5 minutes before serving.

5.78 Wild Rice With Vegetables

Ingredients

1⅓ cups wild rice

2 teaspoons olive oil

2 medium onions, finely diced (about 12 ounces)

2 medium carrots, finely diced (about 6 ounces)

3 large celery stalks, finely diced (about 6 ounces)

1 garlic clove, minced

4 cups vegetables stock

2 tablespoons minced fresh parsley

Salt and pepper to taste

Cooking Instructions

Rinse the rice well and drain. Heat the oil in a deep pan over high heat. Add the onions, carrots, celery, and garlic, and sauté for 2 minutes. Add the rice and sauté for 1 minute. Add the stock and parsley, and bring to a boil. Cover, reduce heat, and cook until tender (approximately 45 minutes but it may depend of the type of rice you use. For best results, see package instructions). Season with salt and pepper and remove from heat. If necessary, strain and serve immediately.

5.79 ROASTED PUMPKIN

You can also use the cooked pumpkin to make apurée or soup. Thin out with low-fat milk until the necessary consistency is reached. You can also use the cooked pumpkin as a base for dips or as a dessert base.

Ingredients

3 pounds sugar pumpkin

1 tablespoon grapeseed oil

Pumpkin pie spice mix

Salt and pepper to taste

Cooking Instructions

Cut open the pumpkin, remove seeds and clean the inside with a spoon. Brush oil inside the cavity, season to taste, and place opening side down on a baking sheet. Roast for 30 to 45 minutes or until tender. Cut out and sprinkle with a little pumpkin pie spices before serving.

5.80 Orange-Glazed Carrots

Ingredients

1 tablespoon grapeseed oil

1 small sweet onion, diced (about 4 ounces)

6 cups baby carrots (about 1½ pounds)

1 teaspoon honey

1½ cups orange juice

3 tablespoons minced fresh parsley

Salt and pepper to taste

Cooking Instructions

Heat the oil in a saucepan over high heat. Add the onions and carrots, and brown slightly. Add the honey and just enough orange juice to cover the vegetables (about 1½ cups). Bring to a boil and cook over medium heat until the liquid is almost completely evaporated. Add the chopped parsley and season lightly with salt and pepper.

5.81 EGGPLANT MEDITERRANEAN STYLE

Ingredients

2 small eggplants, both ends trimmed (about 1 pound)

1 tablespoon paprika

1 tablespoon ground ginger

1 tablespoon garlic powder

1 teaspoon coriander

1 teaspoon cumin

½ teaspoon cayenne pepper

¼ teaspoon ground thyme

¼ teaspoon ground oregano

2 tablespoons olive oil

Salt

Cooking Instructions

Cut eggplant slices lengthwise and arrange on baking sheet. Mix all the spices together. On both sides of the eggplant slices, brush olive oil, season with salt, and sprinkle the prepared spices. Preheat the broiler or barbecue. Broil or grill until golden brown, about 2 minutes per side.

5.82 PORCINI MUSHROOMS PROVENCE STYLE

Ingredients

2 pounds Porcini mushrooms

3 tablespoons olive oil

2 tablespoons minced garlic

½ teaspoon minced fresh thyme

2 tablespoons minced fresh parsley

1 tablespoon minced fresh basil

Salt and pepper to taste

Cooking Instructions

Clean the porcini by brushing off the dirt and then wiping them carefully with a damp cloth. Slice the mushrooms and set aside.

Heat the oil in a large nonstick pan over medium heat. Add the garlic and cook for 15 seconds. Add the mushrooms, thyme, and sauté for 2 to 3 minutes. Add the parsley and basil, and season with salt and pepper. Cook for 2 minutes more and serve immediately.

5.83 POTATO PARSNIP PUREE

Ingredients

8 medium potatoes (about 3 pounds)

1 large parsnip (about 6 ounces)

3 large garlic cloves, peeled

½ cup vegetable stock

1 tablespoon olive oil

1 tablespoon minced fresh parsley

1 tablespoon minced fresh chives

Salt and pepper to taste

Cooking Instructions

Peel and quarter the potatoes and parsnip. Place them in a deep pan and add enough cold water to cover. Add the garlic cloves, ¼ teaspoon salt, and bring to a boil over high heat. Cook until cooked through, about 20 to 25 minutes. Strain through a sieve, reserving the cooking liquid, and puree with a potato masher. Add the vegetable stock and oil, and mix briefly. If too thick, add a little of the reserved cooking liquid to get to the right consistency. Mix in the parsley and chives, season with salt and pepper, and serve immediately.

5.84 Spinach with Pine Nuts and Raisins

Ingredients

2 tablespoons grapeseed oil

1/3 cup plump raisins

1 tablespoon pine nuts

2 pounds fresh spinach, washed and patted dry

Salt and pepper to taste

Cooking Instructions

Heat the oil in a nonstick pan over medium heat. Add the raisins, pine nuts, and sauté for 1 minute. Add the spinach and sauté very briefly. Season with salt and peper and serve immediately. The spinach should be barely wilted to avoid turning to mush.

5.85 BROCCOLI AND PISTACHIO VINAIGRETTE

Ingredients

1 teaspoon Dijon mustard

1 tablespoon minced shallots

1 teaspoon minced garlic

4 tablespoons olive oil

3 tablespoons lemon juice

1 tablespoon minced fresh parsley

Florets from 2½ large heads broccoli (about 1½ pounds)

4 teaspoons chopped pistachios

Salt and pepper to taste

Cooking Instructions

In a bowl, mix the mustard, shallot, garlic, oil, lemon juice, and parsley, and season with salt and pepper.

Preheat a steamer. Add the broccoli and cook for 2 to 3 minutes or to desired doneness. Heat the vinaigrette in a pan over medium heat until warm. Transfer the cooked broccoli to a bowl. Pour the warmed vinaigrette and toss. Sprinkle the pistachios and serve immediately.

5.86 Olive Paste and Red Bell Pepper Bruschetta

Ingredients

2 large red bell peppers (about one pound)

1½ cups pitted black olives

2 ounces capers, rinsed and pat-dried

4 large garlic cloves, minced

½ lemon, juiced

½ cup olive oil

2 ounces anchovy fillets, rinsed and pat-dried

1 French baguette

Salt and pepper to taste

Cooking Instructions

Preheat the broiler. Place the red bell peppers on a baking sheet and char on all sides. If you have a gas stovetop, you may char the bell peppers over the flames. Once blackened on all sides, place in a paper bag and seal. Let stand for 10 minutes. Peel and seed the bell peppers. Remove ribs and slice into ½-inch wide strips.

In a food processor, puree the olives, capers, garlic, oil, lemon juice, and anchovy fillets. The paste should be smooth and spreadable. If it is too thick, add a little more olive oil. Season with salt and pepper and refrigerate for 30 minutes.

With a serrated knife, cut the baguette into ¾-inch-thick slices. Place the slices on a baking sheet. Broil on both sides until golden brown. Cool before use.

Spread some olive paste on each bread slice and top with 1 slice of red bell-pepper. Serve immediately.

5.87 FRENCH CRÊPES

Ingredients

1 cup whole wheat flour

2 extra-large eggs

1 tablespoon sugar

2 tablespoons unsalted butter, melted

2 tablespoons vanilla extract

Pinch salt

1 cup milk

Grapeseed oil

Cooking Instructions

Place the flour in a bowl. Blend in the eggs, sugar, butter, vanilla, and salt. Slowly, whisk in the milk. Let the batter rest for 30 minutes. Before use, add a little water to thin out the batter (you should aim for a thinner consistency than pancakes).

Heat a nonstick pan or crêpe pan over medium heat. Soak a small piece of paper towel with 1 teaspoon grapeseed oil and swirl quickly over the pan. Add enough batter and swirl to cover the entire bottom. Cook until golden brown and turn over. Cook until slightly golden brown. Add filling (see this page) or remove from pan and set aside for later use.

5.88 APPLE FILLING FOR CRÊPES

Ingredients

5 large apples

¼ cup lemon juice

½ cup plus 2 tablespoons apple butter

¼ cup plus 1 tablespoon walnuts

¼ cup plus 1 tablespoon raisins

10 crêpes (see this page)

Cinnamon to taste

Cooking Instructions

Peel and slice the apples. Place them immediately in lemon juice to prevent browning. Poach the apples in the lemon juice plus enough water to cover them halfway (heightwise) and a little cinnamon. Cook until the apples are just barely tender. Remove from heat, drain, and set aside.

Spread 1 tablespoon apple butter on a warm crêpe. Add 2 ounces apples in the center. Sprinkle 1½ teaspoons walnuts, 1½ teaspoons raisins, and cinnamon. Fold each side over the center and continue to cook for a minute. Repeat with remaining crêpes. Serve immediately.

5.89 STRAWBERRY FILLING FOR CRÊPES

Ingredients

10 tablespoons blackcurrant or boysenberry preserves

1⅓ pounds strawberries, trimmed and thinly sliced

10 crêpes (see this page)

Cooking Instructions

Spread 1 tablespoon preserves evenly on a warm crêpe. Add 2 ounces strawberries in the center. Fold each side over the center and continue to cook for a minute. Repeat with remaining crêpes. Serve immediately.

5.90 CHERRY COMPOTE WITH VANILLA ICE CREAM

Ingredients

1 pound English or Montmorency cherries

3 ounces sugar

½ cup water

¼ teaspoon almond extract

¼ teaspoon arrowroot or cornstarch mixed with a little water

2 cups low-fat vanilla ice cream

Cooking Instructions

Remove cherry pits and stalks. Place the cherries in a pan, add the water, sugar, almond extract, and bring to a boil over medium heat. Simmer for 10 minutes. Thicken with the arrowroot mixture and remove from heat. Cool and refrigerate. Divide among four bowls and top with the ice cream.

5.91 Chocolate Cake with Raspberry Coulis

Ingredients

For the cake:

6 large eggs, seperated

½ cup plus 1 tablespoon sugar

8 ounces bittersweet chocolate, chopped

½ cup unsalted butter

2 tablespoons raspberry liquor

For the coulis:

2 cups fresh raspberries

1 teaspoon lemon juice

¼ cup maple syrup

Cooking Instructions

For the cake: Preheat the oven to 350°F. Grease the bottom and sides of 9-inch cake pan. Line the bottom with parchment paper.

In a mixer, whisk the egg yolks with the ½ cup sugar until pale in color and set aside. In a double boiler, melt the chocolate and butter over low heat. Mix until well incorporated. Remove from the double boiler, blend in the raspberry liquor, and let cool a bit. Add the chocolate mixture to the egg yolks mixture and mix well. Whip the egg whites until soft peaks form. Add the 1 tablespoon sugar and continue to beat until the stiff peaks form. Carefully fold in one-third of the egg whites into the cake batter. Fold in another one-third and then the final one-third. Do not overmix, as the egg whites may collapse and your cake will be flat and heavy.

Carefully pour the batter into the prepared pan and bake for 30 minutes or until a tooth pick inserted in the center comes out dry. Transfer to a cooling rack and let cool for 10 minutes. Remove pan and discard the parchment paper. Let cool completely.

For the coulis: In a blender, mix the raspberries. Add the juice and maple syrup. Mix until smooth, and thin out with a little water, if necessary. Pass through a sieve to remove seeds. Refrigerate and serve cold, on the side, with the chocolate cake.

5.92 ORANGE SALAD WITH CHAMPAGNE

Ingredients

8 large oranges

3 tablespoons orange blossoms honey

1 teaspoon coriander seeds (optional)

1½ cups water

1 cup dry Champagne

2 tablespoons Grand Marnier or orange liqueur

Cooking Instructions

Peel and slice the oranges using a paring knife. Do not leave any white membranes on the oranges, as they have a bitter taste.

Heat the honey, coriander, if using, and water in a saucepan over high heat for approximately 10 minutes to end up with 1 cup. Strain into a large bowl and set aside to cool. Mix in the Champagne and liqueur. Add the orange slices and refrigerate at least an hour before serving.

5.93 OATMEAL COOKIES

Ingredients

7 ounces almond meal

¾ cup brown sugar

1½ teaspoons baking powder

¾ teaspoon baking soda

¼ teaspoon salt

1 extra large egg

2 ounces apricot preserves

1 cup Old Fashioned

Quaker Oats

2 ounces unsalted butter

Cooking Instructions

Preheat the oven to 350°F. Prepare a couple of cookie sheets covered with a silpat mat or parchment paper. Mix the almond meal, brown sugar, baking powder, baking soda, and salt. Blend in the egg and the preserves. Melt the butter and let cool for a minute. Add the oats to the almond mixture and mix well. Add the melted butter. Scoop out the dough with a #30 scoop (about 1 ounce cookie) onto the cookie sheet, placing the mounds 3 inches apart to allow for spreading. Refrigerate for 30 minutes. Flatten the dough slightly with your palm and bake for 12 minutes or until golden brown. Let cool in the pan before transferring to a cooling rack.

This type of cookie will be moist. Don't store for more than 2 days at room temperature. It absorbs moisture quickly and can become very soggy. The best way to store them would be to freeze immediately after they cool down. Defrost at room temperature as needed or quickly defrost in the microwave for 5 to 7 seconds.

You may add ½ cup of raisins, dried fruits, coconut, chocolate chips, chopped dates, nuts, or a combination of various ingredients. Remember, any of these ingredients will add calories to the original recipe.

You may also add 1 teaspoon cinnamon and/or ½ teaspoon allspice.

5.94 POMEGRANATE AND STRAWBERRY PARFAIT

Ingredients

1½ cups strawberries

2 ounces pure acai, no sugar added

1 teaspoon vanilla extract

1 cup low-fat Greek yogurt

2 tablespoons pomegranate seeds

Cooking Instructions

Mix the strawberries with vanilla extract and acai. Marinade for 30 minutes. Spoon half the fruit mixture into four parfait glasses. Top with yogurt and finish with the berries. Sprinkle with the pomegranate seeds and serve immediately.

5.95 STRAWBERRIES WITH SPICY RED WINE

Ingredients

4 teaspoons walnuts

4 large apples

9 teaspoons pomegranate preserves

4 tablespoons pomegranate juice

4 tablespoons pomegranate seeds

Cooking Instructions

In a saucepan, combine the wine, honey, vanilla, peels, and peppercorns. Bring to a boil over high heat. Continue to boil until the wine is reduced by half. Remove from heat and strain, discarding the solids.

Place the strawberries in a bowl and pour the hot wine over. Mix well and let cool. Refrigerate for at least 2 hours. Serve cold.

5.96 YOGURT WITH PRUNES

Ingredients

1 pound prunes,3 ounces sugar

12 ounces water

16 ounces low-fat Greek yogurt

Cooking Instructions

Soak the prunes in water for two hours. Transfer to a pan, add the sugar, and bring to a simmer over

medium heat. Reduce heat and continue to cook for
1 hour. Remove from heat and let cool. Refrigerate
until cold.

Divide the yogurt into four serving bowls, top with
the prunes, and serve immediately.

5.97 APPLE AND PEAR MINESTRONE

Ingredients

1 medium apple, brunoise (about 5 ounces)

1 medium pear, brunoise (about 5 ounces)

¾ cup jasmine green tea (or your favorite)

1½ teaspoons honey

½ teaspoon pumpkin pie spices

1 small ginger root, minced

½ teaspoon lemon zest

½ teaspoon grapeseed oil

Cooking Instructions

Heat the oil in a deep saucepan over high heat. Add the apple and sauté for two minutes. Add the pear, spices, ginger, lemon zest, and sauté another minute. Add the green tea and bring to a boil. Remove from heat and transfer to a serving bowl. Cool at room temperature. Refrigerate for an hour or, even better, overnight to allow flavors to emerge. Serve cold.

5.98 BAKED APPLES WITH POMEGRANATE PRESERVES

Ingredients

4 teaspoons walnuts

4 large apples

9 teaspoons pomegranate preserves

4 tablespoons pomegranate juice

4 tablespoons pomegranate seeds

Cooking Instructions

Preheat the broiler. Cover the bottom of a baking sheet with parchment paper. Add the walnuts and broil until slightly browned. Remove from the sheet, cool, and chop.

Preheat the oven to 400°F.

Wash and core the apples, being careful not to break through the bottom of the apples. Place them in a baking pan that is just the right size to keep the apples close to each other. Put 1 teaspoon of pomegranate preserves in the cavity of each apple. Pour 1 tablespoon of pomegranate juice into the cavity of each apple. Add a little hot water to the pan (about ¼ inch high). Cover the pan with aluminum foil and bake for 20 minutes. Remove foil and baste with the pan liquids. Continue baking uncovered for 4 to 5 minutes. If necessary, add a little more water to avoid burning.

Place each apple in a serving dish. Scrape particles from the pan and transfer the liquid to a saucepan. Blend the liquid with the remaining pomegranate preserves and bring to boil over high heat. Pour over the apples, sprinkle the walnuts, pomegranate seeds, and serve immediately.

5.99 Baked Apples with Toasted Walnuts

Ingredients

4 teaspoons walnuts

4 apples

9 teaspoons orange preserves

4 tablespoons Chardonnay (with apple and citrus tones)

Cooking Instructions

Preheat the broiler. Cover the bottom of a baking sheet with parchment paper. Add the walnuts and toast until slightly browned. Remove the walnuts from the sheet, cool, and chop.

Lower the oven to 400°F. Wash and core the apples, being careful not to break through the bottom of the apples. Place them in a baking pan that is just the right size to keep the apples close to each other. Put 1 teaspoon of preserves in the cavity of each apple. Pour one tablespoon of wine over the cavity of each apple. Add a little hot water in the pan, about ¼ inch high. Then cover the pan with aluminum foil and bake for 20 minutes. Remove cover and baste with the liquid in the pan. Continue baking uncovered for 4 to 5 minutes. If necessary, add a little more water.

Place each apple in a dessert dish. Scrape particles from the pan and transfer along with the remaining liquids to a saucepan. Blend the liquid with the remaining 5 teaspoons preserves and bring to a boil over high heat. Pour over the apples, sprinkle the walnuts, and serve immediately.

5.100 DATES WITH ALMONDS

Ingredients

8 dates

4 tablespoons almonds

Cooking Instructions

Divide the dates and almonds in 4 dessert plates and serve immediately.

5.101 FRUIT JUICE POPSICLES

Ingredients

¾ cup pomegranate juice

½ cup orange juice

4 ounces acai, no sugar added

Cooking Instructions

Mix the juices in a blender. Transfer to popsicle molds and freeze.

5.102 MELON SOUP

Ingredients

2 cantaloupes (about 4 cups flesh)

2 tablespoons honey (warmed in the microwave for about 10 seconds)

4 mint leaves

1 lemon, juiced

Cooking Instructions

Cut the cantaloupes in half. Remove all the seeds. Spoon out the flesh and place in a blender. Add the honey, mint, and lemon juice. Puree and refrigerate. Serve cold.

5.103 Papaya Brulée

Ingredients

2 small papayas

4 teaspoons brown sugar

Cooking Instructions

Preheat the broiler. Cut the papayas in half and remove the seeds. Spread the sugar over each half. Place under the broiler and grill until caramelized. This is pretty quick, so keep an eye on the papayas. It will take approximately 1 minute.

5.104 Peach with Apricot Coulis

Ingredients

4 peaches

12 apricots

1 tablespoon honey

1 teaspoon lemon juice

1 rosemary branch

4 teaspoons almonds

5.105 COOKING INSTRUCTIONS

Cut apricots in half and remove pits. Place the apricots in a pan. Add ½ cup water, honey, rosemary, lemon juice, and bring to a boil. Reduce heat, cover, and simmer for ten minutes. Purée in a blender and transfer to a serving bowl. Let cool and refrigerate. Peel and cut the peaches in half. Place the peach halves in a serving platter, drizzle with some apricot sauce and the almonds. Serve with the remaining apricot sauce on the side.

5.106 POACHED PEARS WITH BLACK MUSCAT

Ingredients

½ lemon

½ orange

2 large ripe Bosc pears

12 ounces black Muscat

1 cinnamon stick

1 teaspoon vanilla extract

1 teaspoon ground cardamom

1½ tablespoons honey

Cooking Instructions

Remove a large piece of lemon peel from the lemon and set aside. Juice the lemon and set aside. Remove a large piece of orange peel from the orange and set aside. Juice the orange and set aside.

Peel, halve, and core the pears. Place them in a bowl and add the reserved lemon juice. Mix well to prevent browning.

In a saucepan, combine the wine, peels, orange juice, cinnamon stick, vanilla, honey, and cardamom. Bring to a simmer over medium heat. Add the pears with the lemon juice, and simmer until tender when pierced with a knife, 25 to 30 minutes. Remove the pears and set aside in a serving bowl. Reduce the wine until it thickens like syrup to concentrate the flavors. Cool slightly, pass through a sieve, and add the sauce to the pears. Refrigerate and serve cold.

5.107 WINTER FRUIT SALAD

Ingredients

1 small banana, sliced

6 ounces berries or mango

1 apple, diced

6 ounces grapes

1 orange, peeled and segmented

¼ cup pomegranate seeds

2 tablespoons lemon juice

Cooking Instructions

Blend all the fruits in a large bowl. Mix in the lemon juice, pomegranate seeds, and refrigerate until use.

6 CONCLUSION

Hyperthyroidism occurs when the thyroid gland overproduces thyroid hormone. This can speed up metabolism and cause many body-wide symptoms, including feeling nervous and fatigued and having hand tremors and an irregular heartbeat. A variety of factors can cause hyperthyroidism.

Prompt diagnosis and treatment of hyperthyroidism can return thyroid hormone to appropriate levels, relieve the symptoms, and prevent long-term health problems.

With regular medical care and compliance with their treatment plan, many people with this condition live active, healthy lives.